Prescriptions

for

Independence

Working with
Older People who are
Visually Impaired

Nora Griffin-Shirley
Gerda Groff

AFB

PRESS

NEW YORK

6-13-97

Prescriptions for Independence: Working with Older People Who Are Visually Impaired is copyright © 1993 by
AFB Press
American Foundation for the Blind
15 West 16th Street, New York, NY 10011

97 96 95 94 93   5 4 3 2 1

Printed in the United States of America

Library of Congress Cataloging-in-Publication Data

Griffin-Shirley, Nora, 1954-
   Prescriptions for independence: working with older people who are visually
impaired / Nora Griffin-Shirley and Gerda Groff.
      p.   cm.
   ISBN 0-89128-244-0
   1. Visually handicapped aged—life skills guides.   2.   Life skills
—Study and teaching.   I. Groff, Gerda, 1940-   . II. Title.
HV1597.5.G74 1993
362.4'048—dc20   93-32826
                                                              CIP

CONTENTS

FOREWORD

By now, everyone has heard or read about the graying of America, but not everyone may be aware that as our population ages, it is developing a higher incidence of visual impairment. Increasing numbers of persons will be not just older but older and visually impaired. We at the American Foundation for the Blind want to make certain that these individuals and the people who live and work with them know that life after vision loss does not correspond to myths and stereotypes but can be independent, satisfying, and as full of one's interests and pursuits as before.

Prescriptions for Independence: Working with Older People Who Are Visually Impaired has been designed to provide comprehensive information in a clear and readable way so that visually impaired people, their friends and families, and those who work with them have simple suggestions within easy reach. Readers will find that most people who are visually impaired do have usable vision and do not require special assistance, but they will also find what they need to know about common forms of visual impairment and adaptations and information that are useful to some visually impaired people in daily life. Anyone who knows an older person with a vision loss will find that *Prescriptions for Independence* is a valuable resource for the pursuit of independent living.

Carl R. Augusto
President and Executive Director
American Foundation for the Blind

INTRODUCTION

If you work with older people—whether in a community center, a senior citizens' center, a retirement community, or a residential facility—this book is intended for you. We know, from the work you have chosen, that you are a caring individual, and we also know that some of the people you serve may require some special assistance.

Although you may not yet have noticed it, we are certain that a number of visually impaired people take part in your programs because statistics show a close correlation between age and vision problems. Today, more than 80 percent of people with visual impairments in the United States are over age 65. And with the rapid growth of the senior population, the number of visually impaired older persons in this country is certain to increase over the next decade.

It is easy not to notice the visual impairment of some older persons because these people do not stand out in any way. In spite of their vision loss, they are able to manage effectively without any help from you. They get around, dress, clean house, read, write, and perform other daily activities just about as well as everyone else. It is important to remember that the great majority of visually impaired people do have some usable vision.

Others, however, can benefit from learning techniques that can help them do their daily tasks. They can also benefit from knowing how to adapt their living quarters to make them both safe and efficient. They need to be aware of resources, such as agencies for visually impaired persons, support groups, and services, that can help to make their lives more comfortable and your services and programs more effective and efficient.

We call the techniques, the adaptations, and the resources "prescriptions for independence," because they allow people to do just that—remain independent. Like everyone else, older people cherish their independence, and visually impaired older people are no different from their peers in this regard. They want to do things on their own. They want to be able to participate in the programs you run, and with a little help from you, they can. In this book, we show you how to provide that help.

First, we set the stage: We tell you about the basic types of visual impairment among elderly people, demonstrate how you can help a newly diagnosed person adapt to his or her vision loss, and dispel all-too-prevalent myths about visual impairment. Then we teach you various techniques that you, in turn, can teach visually impaired older people. These are methods for

- moving around safely
- reading and writing

- eating
- handling money
- telling time
- performing personal care routines.

We also show you how you can be aware of safety factors in your own center or facility and how you can work to change situations that need correction.

Finally, we discuss some of the ways that you can extend your work on behalf of older adults who are visually impaired by starting a support group, working with volunteers, and giving families the information they need.

The activities we suggest in this book are important for several reasons:
- They will enhance the quality of the lives of the visually impaired older people you know.
- They will enable visually impaired older people to participate fully in your programs.
- They will help to demonstrate your facility's responsiveness to the Americans with Disabilities Act of 1990, which protects the civil rights of all disabled people, including those who are visually impaired.
- They will help make your facility safer for visually impaired persons and everyone else.
- They will help visually impaired people in your programs remain independent and thereby reduce the time that the staff spends in helping them.

Much of the material in *Prescriptions for Independence* is exciting to learn and to put into practice. At least we feel that way, even after many years of working in the field, and we hope that you will, too. We realize, though, that for many of you, absorbing these techniques and teaching them will be a journey into unknown territory. Let us assure you that it will not take you long to feel at home. You will find that nothing in this book is difficult to understand or to explain to those you are helping. No one expects you to take the place of trained specialists in the area of blindness and visual impairment. Instead, we simply offer ways of expanding the horizons of your program.

Prescriptions for Independence was originally developed as a series of workshops for people who work as nurses' aides in residential facilities. The response was so positive that we decided to adapt it to reach a broader audience. Now, we believe, we have organized the material so it can be useful to everyone who works with elderly persons—professionals, administrators, other staff members, and volunteers—in short, *you,* wherever you fit into the picture.

As you read, you will notice that we attempt to guide you carefully each step of the way, using the actions of people like yourself in similar situations as teaching examples. We want you to understand how our techniques can be applied in real life. We want to encourage you to make them a part of your life—and a part of the lives of the visually impaired people you work with.

You can use this book by yourself or in a group. If you are an administrator, you can plan training sessions based on some of the chapters. Note that the learning exercises for volunteers, presented in Chapter 10, can also be used as addenda to the techniques taught in Chapters 4-8, depending on the amount of time that you and your colleagues have available for group practice.

In short, you can use *Prescriptions for Independence* in a number of ways. Only you know the requirements of your job and the needs of your facility. We can assure you, though, that if you want to make visually impaired elderly people feel that they are truly a part of your program, this book is the right Rx for you.

ACKNOWLEDGMENTS

Prescriptions for Independence is the result of an evolutionary process. To meet the needs of members of the expanding older population who are visually impaired, the American Foundation for the Blind (AFB) received a grant from the Jessie Ball duPont Religious, Charitable and Educational Fund to develop a training curriculum for staff of personal care homes, retirement centers, and nursing homes on how to assist residents with visual impairments. As part of this process, an advisory committee was established to guide the development and evaluation of the curriculum, which was then field-tested in 13 facilities in Georgia, with more than 500 people participating in the training sessions. Based on the feedback from the advisory committee and the persons participating in the field test, the original materials were revised, and they were subsequently further transformed from a training manual into the materials you see now.

The authors would therefore like to thank the following people and organizations that participated in this process:

The Jessie Ball duPont Religious, Charitable and Educational Fund, which provided the funding for the development of the material originally used in training workshops for nursing assistants in residential facilities in Georgia.

The members of the project advisory committee for giving so generously of their time: Tom Dennis, Georgia Division of Rehabilitation Services; Patrice Ernest, Atlanta Regional Commission; Clyde Harrison, Clairmont Oaks; Roy Herzbach, Long Term Health Care Ombudsman Program of Metro Atlanta; Mary McKinnon, Georgia State University Gerontology Center; Pat McMurray, A. G. Rhodes Nursing Home; Elizabeth F. Mistretta, Georgia State University School of Nursing; Ann Reneau, Georgia Nursing Home Association; Linda Smith, Heather House; Andrea Whittaker, Canterbury Court; and Ellyn Yeager, Atlanta Area Chapter, Alzheimer's Association.

The facilities and organizations of metropolitan Atlanta that graciously participated in the field testing: Atlanta Area Chapter, Alzheimer's Association; Bonterra Nursing Center; Campbell Stone North Apartments; Canterbury Court; Clairmont Oaks; Crestview Nursing Home; DeKalb County Housing Authority; Georgia Association of Homes and Services for the Aging; Georgia Association of Personal Care Homes; Georgia Nursing Home Association; Georgia State University and Atlanta Regional Commission's Continuing Education Program for Church, Synagogue, and Community Agencies; Home Place Personal Care Home; Home Providers United; Jewish Home; Jewish Tower; Lenbrook Square; Long Term Health Care Ombudsman Program of Metro Atlanta; Manor Care; Mountain View Personal Care Home; Neighbor Senior Center; Rosemaude Personal Care Home; and

Sue's Benevolence Personal Care Home; as well as the Broward Center for the Blind in Fort Lauderdale, Florida.

The staff of the National Program Associates Department of AFB for sharing their expertise and support, particularly Alberta Orr, program associate specializing in aging, and Lynne Luxton, former program associate specializing in rehabilitation teaching and independent living.

The staff of AFB Press, specifically Natalie Hilzen, managing editor, books and pamphlets; Mary Ellen Mulholland, director; Sharon Shively, assistant editor; and Carol Wallace, executive secretary; as well as Jean Arbeiter, who helped refashion the manuscript into its present form.

Our colleagues who worked with us at the Southeast Regional Center of AFB in Atlanta: Oraien E. Catledge, former regional specialist in aging, now retired, for getting the ball rolling; Elizabeth Burson, project assistant, who kept all the balls in play; and Elnora C. Pierce, project secretary, who wrapped it all up with a polished, typed manuscript.

PRESCRIPTIONS FOR INDEPENDENCE

CHAPTER 1

RECOGNIZING VISION PROBLEMS

Congratulations on your commitment to helping older people with vision loss. Most of these people, as you will see, do not have severe vision loss and can manage well on their own with nothing more than supportive awareness by you. Others can benefit from learning techniques—which will be described later in this book—for getting around, reading, writing, eating, caring for themselves, and caring for their living quarters. By imparting these techniques, you can make a big difference in the quality of an older person's life, as well as your own. And, by being aware of safety factors, you can make your facility a warm and welcoming place for all older people who are visually impaired.

But to be of assistance, you first need to know about the five major conditions that cause vision loss—also called visual impairment—among elderly persons and the effects of these conditions. Some may be familiar to you, whereas others may not. Here are a few facts about each condition:

Age-related maculopathy, which is also called macular degeneration, is the leading cause of severe vision loss in people over age 65. This progressive condition impairs central vision, which is the vision we need to read, write, and recognize faces. As a result, people have to depend on their peripheral, or side, vision to get around and perform tasks. There is no cure for most cases of age-related maculopathy, but some cases, if caught early, can be treated with laser surgery.

Cataract is a clouding of the lens of the eye, which is normally transparent. It varies in size and may cause little trouble in some people, but serious blurring of the field of vision in others. People with extensive cataracts in both eyes may see only shapes and bright colors. Sometimes the condition can be corrected by surgery in which the lens of the eye is replaced by an artificial lens. Or, contact lenses or eyeglasses are prescribed.

Diabetic retinopathy, which affects only people with diabetes, is damage to the blood vessels behind the eye. Diabetic retinopathy can affect the entire field of vision, and blind spots are common. If caught early, this condition can be treated with laser surgery.

Glaucoma is an increase in pressure in the eye because of the buildup of fluid. In the early stages, there are no changes in vision, but in advanced stages peripheral vision is damaged, resulting in tunnel vision. Discovered early, glaucoma can be treated with eye drops or oral medication.

Hemianopsia, which often occurs as the result of a stroke, is obstructed vision in the right or left side or the top or bottom of the visual field.

The Importance of Vision Checkups

Since some vision problems are preventable, one of the most valuable things you can do is to urge older people to have regular eye examinations. Such examinations are available from an ophthalmologist, a physician who diagnoses and treats eye conditions, or an optometrist, a professional who can diagnose eye conditions and prescribe corrective lenses.

Another thing you can do is to ask your facility to arrange for annual on-site vision screenings. These screenings can be set up by contacting an ophthalmologist in your area; a local chapter of the National Society to Prevent Blindness; or a local chapter of the Delta Gamma Foundation, an organization that funds such screenings as part of its mission (see Resources at the back of this book for more information). You or another staff member may even want to learn how to perform such screenings yourself.

Listening for Vision Problems

You may work with elderly people whose vision problems have already been diagnosed. In fact, they may well tell you about their limitations and suggest ways in which you can be of help. Others, however, may suspect that they have visual difficulties, but hold back from admitting that they may have them. Or they may view the problem as just one more condition that cannot be helped when one gets on in years. But often, something *can* be done, which is why anyone who works with older people should be alert for signs of vision loss.

Sometimes such signs are revealed by what people say. For example, Mr. Gomez told Leslie, the art counselor at his senior citizens' center, that he could not complete a project because "there's a curtain in front of my eyes." Mrs. Taylor, a resident of a long-term care facility, refused to go to the dining room, saying that the bright light hurt her eyes. These statements could have indicated vision problems.

Here are some other things people may say:

- "I see halos or rings around lights." .
- "I have migraine headaches, along with blurry vision."
- "I keep seeing flashes of light."
- "I can't see anything at night."
- "There are spots in front of my eyes."
- "My eyes hurt."
- "I'm seeing double."
- "Everything looks distorted."
- "I can't see very well."
- "I can't see at all."

People with any of these problems should be referred for an eye examination immediately.

Watching for Trouble

Although listening is important, you cannot always wait to be told of difficulties. Since some older people may hesitate to confide in anyone, you also have to be aware of changes in behavior and appearance that could be related to vision.

For example, you may notice that someone who is usually well groomed has started to look sloppy or to wear clothes that do not match. Or, you may find that a person who knows you well has begun to pass you in the hall, as if he or she is no longer able to recognize you. Other signs are being unable to find personal belongings, getting "lost" in areas that should be familiar, and bumping into objects.

In a dining situation, an individual may have trouble identifying what is on the plate. He or she may knock items off the table, spill food on clothing, or simply stop eating to avoid the embarrassment of making a mess.

However, a difficulty with eating is just one of the behaviors that can point to a vision problem. Others include the loss of interest in such activities as being with friends, reading, writing, or watching television.

An apparent personality change is another clue. Mrs. O'Brien, for example, had always been a leader at her community center and an organizer of group events. But gradually, her bubbly personality changed. She became withdrawn and refrained even from activities that used to delight her, like playing the piano. (A list of common behaviors that may indicate vision problems appears in "10 Signs of Vision Loss" in this chapter.)

In addition to behavioral changes, you should also be aware of these physical signs that can indicate a vision problem: a protruding eye, a change in eye color, excessive tearing, and the sudden crossing of an eye.

Bringing up the Issue

If observation leads you to suspect a vision problem, the best thing you can do is to discuss the matter with the person privately and in a gentle manner. You may say something like this: "I notice that you seem to be walking slowly lately. Are you having trouble seeing?" The person may be relieved to have the opportunity to talk about a worrisome situation.

Be sure to allow enough time for the expression of feelings that may have been concealed for some time. Studies show that many older people fear vision loss more than any other condition.

You can allay fears by stressing that most people with vision problems can, with proper diagnosis and training, continue to function independently. You may then want to refer the person to the nearest low vision center for a low vision evaluation, which is an assessment of a person's ability to see.

Low vision centers are staffed by a variety of professionals who act as a team. Ophthalmologists and optometrists diagnose visual impairments and may prescribe eyeglasses and low vision aids, such as magnifiers. Rehabilitation teachers provide instruction in using aids and in performing activities of daily living—cooking, cleaning, dressing, and so forth. Orientation and mobility (O&M) specialists teach people how to move around safely,

---

10 SIGNS OF VISION LOSS

1. Bumping into objects.
2. Moving hesitantly or walking close to the wall.
3. Groping for objects or touching them in an uncertain way.
4. Squinting or tilting the head to see.
5. Requesting additional or different kinds of lighting.
6. Holding books or other reading material close to the face.
7. Dropping food or utensils at mealtimes.
8. Showing difficulty in making out faces or the numbers of rooms or floors.
9. Looking ungroomed or sloppy, with stains on clothing, mismatched clothing, or uncombed hair.
10. Acting confused or disoriented; for example, walking into the wrong room by mistake.

both inside and outside their homes. In short, the staff of a low vision center can do a great deal to foster a person's independence and calm his or her fears.

Low vision centers can frequently be found through local hospitals or university medical centers. The American Foundation for the Blind (AFB) can also provide you with the names of low vision centers near you. Another good source is your local agency for visually impaired persons, which may even run such a center itself. There are also governmental and national agencies that help visually impaired people in various ways. (See "Where to Get Help" in this chapter and the Resources section at the back of this book.)

Thinking about Your Own Thinking

If you want to help visually impaired people, you probably also need to examine your attitudes. Certain beliefs about visual impairment are common in our culture, and even if you are not aware of them, they may be influencing the way you think.

Let us begin the demythologizing process by looking at some commonly held beliefs about older people in general:
- All older people are pretty much alike.
- Mental confusion is inevitable, if you live long enough.
- Intelligence declines with age.
- Most older people have no interest in sexual relations.
- Most older people feel miserable all the time.
- Older people are incapable of change.

Since you work with older people, you know that these beliefs are not true. In fact, research has proved them to be false. Yet they continue to affect the way our society treats older people.

Stereotypes about visual impairment are equally invidious, even though they are not all negative. Some beliefs attribute special powers to visually impaired people, such as being musically inclined, having sharpened remaining senses, or being able to perform supernatural deeds. Others view visual impairment as a punishment for sins and conclude that those who suffer from it ought to be feared and shunned. Yet another set of beliefs portrays people with visual impairments as inevitably unhappy and incapable of doing anything for themselves.

Whether one sees visual impairment as a mystical gift, a punishment, or a condition that ends one's usefulness, all stereotypical thinking is just plain inaccurate. Elderly people with vision loss are human beings who happen to have a problem with their eyesight. All that means is that they may have to do some things differently from people with good vision. They may, for example, need to read large-print books or use special techniques for getting around.

But because some visually impaired persons do things differently does not mean they have to be treated differently. In fact, one of the most helpful things you can do is to treat visually impaired older people just as you do other elderly people. If you find that you can feel the effects of stereotypes you were not aware of, try to keep the following principles in mind:
- Each older person is an individual with needs, interests, and desires, just like you and everyone else.
- There is no need to have different expectations for visually impaired people.
- It is important to learn all you can about services for visually impaired persons.
- Referring people to appropriate services is making a valuable contribution to their lives.

You can make an important contribution by continuing to read this book, by acting on what you learn, and by maintaining the attitude that a person can live independently and fully, even without perfect vision.

Older people who are experiencing vision loss should know about the following agencies and the services they provide:

State vocational rehabilitation agency: Funds counseling, low vision services, rehabilitation services, and vocational services through local agencies for visually impaired people. It emphasizes the provision of services to people with disabilities who have the potential for gainful employment.

State agency for visually impaired persons: Provides services that include O&M and rehabilitation teaching. This type of separate agency for persons with visual impairments does not exist in every state.

Local agency for visually impaired persons: Provides a wide range of rehabilitation services and counseling. Fees can be arranged on a sliding scale.

Low vision center: Provides diagnostic services, prescriptions for low vision aids, and training in how to use the aids.

State office on aging: Administers federal and state funds for services to older people. Also, as required by law, has a program of long-term-care ombudspersons, who are public officials or volunteers who investigate and mediate grievances from residents and work with long-term-care institutions to increase their responsiveness to the rights of elderly people.

Local agency on aging: Contracts with local service providers to deliver such assistance as transportation, telephone contact, home care, escort services, and Meals on Wheels.

Social Security Administration: The federal agency that, in addition to providing social security, provides Supplemental Security Income (SSI) to individuals with limited income and resources. To qualify for SSI, a person must be aged 65 or older or legally blind (see Glossary) or disabled, that is, unable to work because of physical or mental problems, and have a low income, as defined by the SSI program.

Local social services department: Provides information on Medicaid, a state-administered program for people whose income and resources fall below a certain level. Generally, those who are eligible for SSI are also eligible for Medicaid, which helps pay the costs of medical care, hospitalization, and nursing home care.

Local senior citizens' or volunteer center: Provides volunteers to work with or visit older people, including those who are visually impaired.

Listings for federal, state, and local agencies can be found in the government sections of local telephone directories. Information about low vision centers and services can be obtained from state and local agencies for visually impaired persons, and information about local senior citizens' centers can be obtained from local agencies on aging.

CHAPTER 2

HELPING PEOPLE COPE WITH VISION LOSS

Most people who are visually impaired do not experience severe vision loss. But whether their impairment is minor, moderate, or severe, they need to adjust to it.

For some people, adjusting is fairly easy. Others experience psychological effects and may require assistance. Though you should not try to take the place of a professional counselor, there are steps you can take to help.

The first step is to be aware of how people are likely to feel, allowing for the fact that not everyone experiences the same turmoil and emotions. Nonetheless, there are several general phases of adjustment to take into account.

Common Reactions

When people find it difficult to perform customary activities, they may experience *trauma,* a disordered mental state, which may become more acute after their visual problem is diagnosed. The following reactions also usually take place:

- *Shock and denial.* People report feeling numb. They may also travel from doctor to doctor, refusing to believe that the initial diagnosis was correct. For example, Mrs. Gray canceled a trip sponsored by her community center because of an appointment with an ophthalmologist. "This is the fifth eye doctor I've seen in six months," she confided to Elaine, a volunteer. "I'm sure that those other doctors are wrong. I don't feel like my vision has gotten any worse."

- *Anger and/or withdrawal.* People often express anger at their situation or show anger to those who are closest to them. They ask questions like, "Why is this happening to me?" They may withdraw from social activities and close friends. Many feel that they have lost control of their lives. "I planned to travel when I retired," Mrs. Gray said angrily to Elaine a few weeks after her last doctor's appointment. "Now I'm just going to have to sit at home. My dreams have been destroyed!"

- *Succumbing and depression.* People often experience strong grief reactions, including crying and sobbing, along with a recognition of loss. Some talk repeatedly about "the way things used to be" when their sight was better. Mrs. Gray mournfully described the books she loved to read "when I could see."

Gradually, with or without help people may go through the next two phases, in which they resolve their problems and learn how to cope with them:

- **Reassessment and reaffirmation.** People identify their strengths and weaknesses, affirm their belief systems, and start to plan for the future. Mrs. Gray, for example, thought about ways of getting around without having to drive and learned how to take the bus to the community center.
- **Coping and mobilization.** People learn new techniques to keep themselves independent. They focus on what they can do, rather than on the abilities they have lost. Mrs. Gray had difficulty writing, so she started sending taped messages to her granddaughter, Susan. "Susan can't write very well, either. She's too young," Mrs. Gray told Elaine. "What a wonderful time for me to discover the tape recorder."

(For a full description of these reactions, see Tuttle's *Self-Esteem and Adjusting with Blindness,* listed in Resources.)

Facilitating Adjustment

Because each person has a distinct pattern of adjusting to any type of loss, the phases just described are not necessarily sequential, nor is one phase completed because a person seems to have moved on to another one. He or she may shift back and forth among phases several times before achieving a final adjustment.

A person's pattern of adjustment is influenced by both internal and external factors. Internal factors include the person's past history, belief system, and the number and severity of other losses he or she is experiencing. External factors include the attitudes of the person's support network—ophthalmologist or optometrist; family members; friends; and others who see the person regularly, such as yourself. You can assist by being sensitive to the person as an individual and, if possible, by providing guidance appropriate to each phase of the adjustment process.

For example, a newly diagnosed person may not have understood everything the doctor said. If that is the case, you can help him or her make a list of questions for the eye care specialist to answer. Reviewing some of the terminology listed in the Glossary of this book can help. Or you can suggest that the person contact AFB for pamphlets that explain medical terms and available services in simple language. Still another possibility is to suggest that someone accompany the person on the next doctor's visit to help listen to or interpret what is being said.

LISTENING ACTIVELY

As you spend time with someone who is adjusting to vision loss, there are several ways in which you can be supportive. For example, an individual who is experiencing denial may want to tell you about the "misdiagnoses" he or she got from doctors. Listening, though not always easy, can be helpful, since the person will eventually "hear" that the physicians are all saying the same thing. If not, you can point out that, "Dr. Steiglitz and Dr. Henderson appear to have made similar evaluations." Putting it this way, you may be able to encourage the person to accept the truth.

People who are angry may express strong emotions. They may sometimes act in an unacceptable way, such as by verbally attacking others. As an alternative, provide appropriate opportunities for the person to discuss his or her feelings openly or try to engage the person in an activity he or she enjoys. Physical exercise is a particularly good choice. Remember that other people in your program may be troubled by the person's anger. If so, explain that it is only temporary and part of the adjustment process. Point out that by being understanding, they can help the person, as you are attempting to do.

Allow people who may be grieving their loss of vision to express their sadness. Talking does not prolong unhappiness; rather, it may encourage its resolution. As you listen, it is better to avoid saying, "I know how you feel," since none of us really does know what someone may be going through. Instead, think about the losses you have experienced in your own life. If you can share what you felt at those times, you can create a bond of empathy. For example, Mrs. Gray's vision problems began around the time that Elaine's father died. By talking about the way she missed her father, Elaine showed Mrs. Gray that she, too, understood feelings of grief.

People in a reassessment phase need to mobilize their inner resources. They also need to sort out what is really important to them in life. Often they will talk about a number of issues without seeming to come to any conclusion. You can help by summarizing and repeating what someone tells you, as in, "I think I'm hearing you say that your family has become more valuable to you." In this way, you can help the person understand what is going on inside.

ENCOURAGING PROGRESS

You can also strengthen someone's adjustment, coping, and mobilization of resources by encouraging him or her to learn adaptive ways of doing important activities. Explain that rehabilitation teachers and O&M specialists are available to help. The services of these professionals can be obtained through low vision centers, local agencies for people with visual impairments, or state rehabilitation programs (see "Where to Get Help" in Chapter 1.) Assure the person that you will be able to help, too.

Finally, as people learn adaptive methods, be enthusiastic about their progress. If you see them using an optical aid, such as a magnifier, comment on it. If they are enrolled in a rehabilitation program, ask what they are being taught. Mrs. Gray told Elaine that she was learning to cook again. "They showed me a new way of knitting, too," she said; "I'm working on a sweater." Elaine asked to see the knitting project and, a few months later, her interest was rewarded with a new scarf that Mrs. Gray had made for her.

As Mrs. Gray's rehabilitation continued, she became increasingly enthusiastic about the options available to her. "I may not be able to see as well as I used to, but my mind still works," she said to Elaine one day. "I want to know what's happening in the world. I'm going to order a receiver from a radio reading service so I can hear the news read out loud every day." A few weeks later, when Elaine saw Mrs. Gray comfortably listening to the receiver, she realized that the adjustment process was beginning.

As people learn how to cope with their vision problems, you can continue to help by stressing independence as an ongoing goal. If you work in a residential facility, try to make sure that residents with vision loss are encouraged to perform the same activities as everyone else. If you work in a senior citizens' center, make certain that the full program is open to people with vision loss.

People who are visually impaired do not need things done for them. They may only need support in doing things for themselves. They are ready—and able—to get on with their lives on their own.

CHAPTER 3

COMMUNICATING AND ENCOURAGING COMMUNICATION

The four chapters following this one tell you how to teach specific skills to visually impaired people. But to transmit skills, you may first have to know how to talk with older people who have vision problems and often hearing loss as well—a combination of impairments that can all too easily lead to isolation.

Seeing someone withdraw because other people may be awkward about carrying on a conversation is unfortunate and can be avoided. Most visually impaired individuals long for human contact, just like everyone else, and by bearing certain facts in mind, you can talk with them as easily as you can with anyone else.

The Road to Easy Talking

The foundation of communicating with another person is to instill a sense of ease and trust. You can do so if you remember to follow the steps outlined in "Encouraging Relaxed Conversations." In addition, there are some specific techniques that can make conversation with a visually impaired person flow more smoothly.

When you approach a visually impaired person, always announce your name and the names of any other people with you—for example, "Good morning, Mrs. Benson. It's Bill, and this is my friend, Nancy Gold."

Shake the person's hand, if you're meeting him or her for the first time. Then position yourself so that the light falls on your face, which usually makes it easier for the person to see you. Ask the person if there is a place he or she would prefer you to sit. When you sit down, maintain eye contact if possible, even if the person does not see well. If you know which eye or ear is the better one, direct your voice toward that eye or ear. Speak slowly and clearly without shouting.

ENCOURAGING RELAXED CONVERSATIONS

- Hold conversations in a pleasant, quiet environment, when possible.
- Allow plenty of time for the person to understand you and to respond.
- Listen as well as talk.
- Use body language—gestures and facial expressions—to help get your points across.
- Be patient and flexible in your expectations.

In short, treat your conversational partner with the same respect you would like accorded to you.

It's all right to describe objects by color or to use words like "look" and "see," even with the minority of visually impaired individuals who have severe vision loss. They will be accustomed to such language.

Remember to describe what is going on around you. For instance, while Bill Hernandez was chatting with Mrs. Benson, the room suddenly became noisy. Bill explained, "They're setting up the chairs for the class," thus allowing Mrs. Benson to become oriented.

If your partner does not understand you, repeat what you said, using different words. When Bill told Mrs. Benson that "the nutrition lecture will begin soon," she looked at him blankly, so he paraphrased: "The talk about which foods are good for you will begin soon." Then he asked Mrs. Benson if she had heard what he had said so he could be sure she got the message.

Be certain not to monopolize the conversation. And, if other people join the discussion, introduce them, explain what is going on, and give them a chance to catch up. Never ask questions of a third party—for example, "Nancy, does Mrs. Benson want a drink?"—when the person with the answer is sitting right next to you. Instead, speak directly: "Would you like a drink, Mrs. Benson?"

When you give directions to a visually impaired person, be specific. "The table is behind you and to your left" is useful; "You'll find the table over there" is not. If you need to convey extensive directions, write them down in large print.

Finally, a word about physical contact: Do not ever touch someone without first asking if it is all right to do so. If it is, go ahead. You will find that many people who are visually impaired appreciate being touched gently on the shoulder, having a hand held, or receiving a hug when they need reassurance—just like everyone else.

Instilling Conversational Confidence

Some visually impaired people hesitate to start a conversation with people who are not visually impaired, even if they feel in need of companionship. For example, Mrs. Benson confided to Bill Hernandez that she thought it was too much trouble for people to bother talking with her.

Bill knew how important it was for Mrs. Benson to keep up her social contacts. He told her that she had a right to talk regularly with others and that everyone wanted to talk to her, too. How could she know, he asked, that people did not want to talk with her if she did not approach them? He encouraged her to try.

Starting a conversation would be easier, Bill pointed out, if Mrs. Benson explained at once that she had some difficulty seeing. That way, she could remind people to identify themselves; to sit near her, rather than talk from afar; and to be sure that their faces were in the light.

With Bill, Mrs. Benson practiced speaking up if she could not hear something or asking for a sentence to be repeated if she did not understand it. She also learned how to move herself and a conversational partner away from a noisy situation so she would not have to shout. In short, she learned how to take control of the conversation.

Nowadays, when Mrs. Benson joins a conversation—as she is increasingly doing—she makes sure to ask one of the participants to catch her up on what is going on.

And, by taking control, Mrs. Benson is also able to get the most out of group "conversations," such as meetings, lectures, and performances, instead of staying away from them. It takes some planning for her to position herself so she can take full advantage of these events. You can pass along the rules she follows to any visually impaired or hearing impaired person:

- If you know that a meeting or lecture will be held in a large room, check to see if arrangements can be made for sound amplification.
- Arrive early at meetings so you can seat yourself close to the speaker or performer.
- Request front-row tickets for plays. Ask if an audiodescription, a taped verbal account of what is happening, will be available. Audiodescription services are also often available to describe the visual aspects and physical action shown in such presentations as films, museum exhibits, television programs, and videotapes. (For more information, see *A Picture Is Worth a Thousand Words for Blind and Visually Impaired Persons Too! An Introduction to Audiodescription,* listed in Resources.)
- If possible, become familiar with the plot of a movie or a play in advance.

Talking with people, taking part in meetings, and enjoying a play or performance are all facets of communication that enhance our humanity and keep us involved in life. Every time you stress the importance of communication and teach the skills that people need to maintain contact with others, you strengthen their ability to be independent. And, by talking regularly with visually impaired people, you enhance your own ability to teach and to learn.

CHAPTER 4

TEACHING BASIC ORIENTATION AND MOBILITY TECHNIQUES

Most of the visually impaired people you work with probably get around capably without using special techniques. In fact, you may not be able to tell from the way they walk or move that they have any vision loss. But some individuals benefit from skills that allow them to move about more safely. These skills are called orientation and mobility (O&M) techniques.

Orientation means using the senses to figure out where one is. For example, a visually impaired person can rely on food odors to tell if a bakery or restaurant or the dining room is nearby. Or, the person can use a change in floor covering from tile to carpet to identify the transition from a hallway to a bedroom.

Mobility means the ability to move from place to place, from home to workplace or shopping area, for example, or simply to be able to walk through one's environment.

Advanced O&M techniques are complicated—they may involve the use of a specialized cane—and must be taught by O&M specialists. You should not get involved in teaching such skills. (In fact, if you do, and an injury results, you could face liability problems.) But there are simple techniques you *can* learn and then teach to people who desire your help. All it takes is a willingness to explore something that is new—and interesting.

Learning to Be a Sighted Guide

Learning how to act as a sighted guide—a gentle, extra hand who facilitates the safe movement of persons with visual impairments—is probably the most basic way to help visually impaired persons when needed. Sighted guide technique can be used in all kinds of situations, but let us begin with guiding someone through an open space, such as an uncrowded room or corridor. (For additional information, the videotape *The Seven-Minute Lesson,* listed in Resources, may be helpful.)

First, remember to ask if your assistance is needed. Most visually impaired people do not need any help, and they may resent having it forced on them. A simple "Can I give you a hand?" or "Do you want any help?" is a good way to find out whether you are wanted. Then, if your help is needed, follow these four basic steps:

- **Step 1.** Touch the person's hand with the back of your hand. Then advise him or her to take hold of your arm just above the elbow or, for more stable support, at the inner elbow (see Figures 1 and 2). If still more support is required, bend your arm at a 90-degree angle to your body and have the person grasp your forearm. Always ask the individual you are helping which technique he or she prefers and try to oblige, if possible.

- **Step 2**. Hold your arm in a relaxed manner, yet close to your body, and tell the person you are helping to do the same (see Figure 3). This stance allows for the

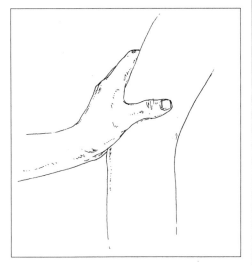

FIGURE 1. Placement of the finger and thumb in the sighted guide technique.

easy interpretation of your movement by the person.

- **Step 3**. Have the person walk about a half step behind you and slightly to the side (see Figure 4). His or her shoulder should be directly behind yours. If you are using the more supportive forearm grasp, the person should be at your side, rather than behind you.
- **Step 4**. Walk at a comfortable pace, neither dragging nor pushing the individual you are helping.

As you walk, keep up a normal conversation, interspersing verbal reminders when necessary. For example, you may say, "We're coming to the end of the corridor." You can also communicate in a nonverbal way, such as by slowing down when approaching an obstacle.

Negotiating Tight Spaces

Spaces are not always open, uncrowded, or easy to navigate. Therefore, you need to know guiding techniques for situations like these:

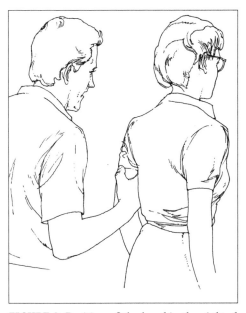

FIGURE 2. Position of the hand in the sighted guide technique.

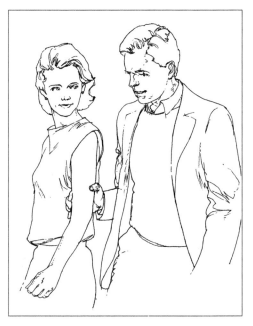

FIGURE 3. Position of the hand and body in the sighted guide technique.

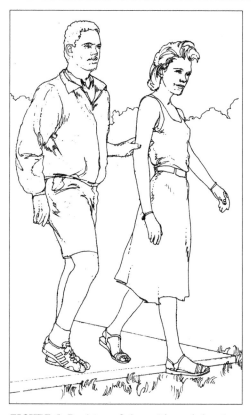

FIGURE 4. Position of the guide and the visually impaired person in the sighted guide technique.

- **Narrow spaces**. To walk between pieces of furniture or through a group of people, move your arm toward the center of your back. This position places the person directly behind you and forces him or her to take smaller steps. Tell the person to extend the arm that is holding yours—"the grasping arm"—to full length so your heels do not get stepped on. If the person is too frail to extend an arm, have him or her stand behind you and put one hand on your waist, if necessary changing the arm used to grasp your arm. Before you reach an open space, turn so you and the person can sidestep through it together.

- **Doorways**. Maneuver so your partner is standing to your side and closest to the door hinges. Have the person hold the door open while you go through first. Then guide him or her through. If the person is not strong enough to hold the door open, hold it open yourself and guide both of you through at the same time or have the person go through ahead of you.

- **Stairways**. Tell your partner whether the stairs go up or down and how many flights there are. Then position the person so he or she can grasp the handrail, if there is one. Walk up or down the stairs in front of the person and one step ahead (see Figure 5). Pause briefly or announce the approach of a landing or the last step.

- **Getting someone seated**. Guide the person to the front of the chair or other seat and describe its position—for example, "You're standing in front of the chair now." For stability, place the person's hand on the chair's back or

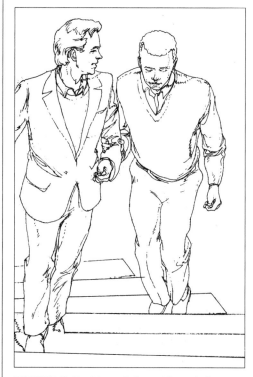

FIGURE 5. Position of the guide and the visually impaired person while climbing stairs.

arm. Have him or her feel the seat with the other hand, turn around, and sit down.

- **Getting someone into a car**. If the person will be opening the car door, point out where the door handle is. Have the person touch the roof of the car with his or her free hand to protect the head while getting in. Depending on the person's vision loss, it may be necessary for you to help support the person by holding his or her arm as he or she steps into the car and sits down. If the person uses a cane, it should be placed near the door so it does not interfere with the driver. Make certain the person closes the car door securely.

Guiding Someone Who Uses Adaptive Equipment

Older people frequently depend on assistance from support canes, walkers, and wheelchairs. Here are a few tips to keep in mind when the people you are helping use such items:

- **Support canes**. Walk on the side away from the cane. If the person needs stronger support, have him or her hold onto your forearm with the hand that is not holding the cane. Adjust your pace to the person's slower pace when he or she is using a cane. Warn of approaching stairs and curbs and allow time for the person to react.
- **Walkers**. Ask the person how he or she would like to be guided. Some people only want to have the environment described to them. Others will ask you to put your hand on one of their hands and walk along with the walker. In either case, keep your pace slow and your steps short. Try to avoid changes in elevation. An individual with a visual impairment may want to go through doorways ahead of you while you hold the door open. Be sure that he or she pauses

with the walker and uses the upper hand and forearm protective technique described in the next section, "Moving about Safely."

- **Wheelchairs**. If you are asked to push someone in a wheelchair, do so, when possible. People who push themselves may want you to guide them by putting your hand on one of their shoulders. Whether you push a wheelchair or walk alongside it, provide information about such structures as stairs and curbs.

Moving about Safely

A sighted guide may not always be available or necessary. All that some people need is to use a safety-bolstering technique that can keep them from bumping into objects or furniture.

If you have observed that someone frequently has such mishaps, suggest that he or she learn two simple means of self-protection. If the person is amenable, you can demonstrate how the methods work. Both rely on holding one forearm away from the body as a gentle buffer against obstacles.

- **METHOD 1: Upper hand and forearm protective technique**. Tell the person to extend the stronger arm straight out ahead, bend and bring it to the opposite shoulder, and hold it about 8 to 10 inches away from the body with the palm turned outward (see Figure 6). Next, have the person lift the arm so it is in front of the face, if possible, as high as the forehead, with the fingers of the hand curled. Advise the individual to keep the fingers and the entire body relaxed while walking.
- **METHOD 2: Lower hand and forearm protective technique**. Tell the person to position the stronger arm comfortably at the belly button, then extend it out about 8 to 10 inches with the palm facing the body. For maximum safety, the other hand can be positioned in the upper

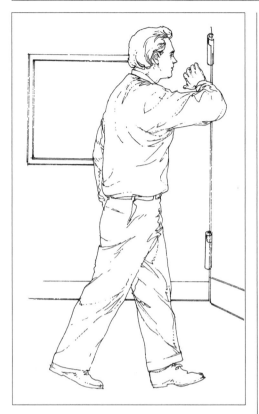

FIGURE 6. Upper hand and forearm protective technique.

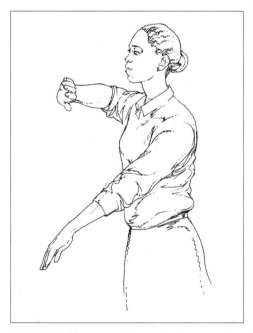

FIGURE 7. Upper and lower body protective techniques.

hand and forearm technique. While walking, body and fingers should be kept relaxed (see Figure 7).

It is a good idea to practice the two methods yourself before teaching them and then to practice with the individual as well. Bear in mind that it can take some time to remember to move about with one's arm extended.

The selection of a method, by the way, should depend, in part, on the height of the hazards one is likely to encounter. Another consideration is the degree of the person's infirmity. You may need to modify these techniques. For example, in the lower hand and forearm protective technique, the person can position his or her arm off center, rather than at the belly button. When you modify a technique, though, be certain not to sacrifice safety.

"Trailing" One's Way

In conjunction with protective techniques, you may want to teach a skill called "trailing." Trailing is a way of moving the fingers along a wall to keep a straight line, to find a door, or to walk through a building. Usually, trailing is done along the right wall of a hallway or room (see Figure 8).

To teach the technique, have the individual do the following:

● Stand parallel to the wall and close to it.
● Touch the wall with the hand nearest to it.
● Cup the fingers slightly for protection and move the backs of the fingers, particularly the knuckles of the index and middle fingers, gently along the wall while walking (see Figure 9).

When the person comes to a doorway, he or she should trail across the opening, taking care not to get off balance or to veer into the room. The upper hand and forearm technique should also be used here to avoid bumping the face against a door frame.

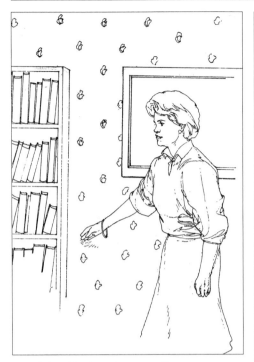

FIGURE 8. Trailing along a wall.

As with the protective methods, trailing takes some practice. So remember to allow plenty of time when you are teaching this technique. Also remember to stay with the person the first few times he or she tries it.

Familiarizing Someone with a Room

Once protective methods and trailing have been mastered, they can be used to

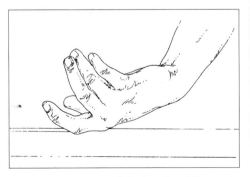

FIGURE 9. Position of the hand and fingers in trailing.

explore new environments. But these skills may not always be sufficient. Sometimes, the assistance of an individual with full vision, such as yourself, will be needed as well.

To be helpful, first imagine yourself walking into a room you have never seen before. You would be able to take in the key aspects—size, function, and decor—with just a glance or two.

You need to realize, however, that some visually impaired people cannot see well enough to learn about a room this way. To master the terrain, they need to have the room presented to them in a step-by-step manner. In short, they need to learn the room-familiarization technique.

You may be able to tell from the way a person moves whether this technique is needed. For example, Lisa Chang, an administrator at a retirement community, noticed that Mr. Bryce, a visually impaired man who had just moved into the community, had difficulty finding his way around. She would have to help him become familiar with various rooms and areas.

Lisa started with the large recreation room, one of the most commonly used areas in the main building. First, she stood with Mr. Bryce in the doorway for a moment or two and told him what the room was used for. Then she asked if there were any objects near the door that would help him to identify the room in the future. Mr. Bryce settled on a brightly colored switchplate that contrasted with the wall. With Lisa's urging, he committed the position of the switchplate to memory.

Lisa advised Mr. Bryce to trail one wall of the room at a time—starting with the right wall—and then return to the entryway. She suggested that he "label" each wall in the room to differentiate it from the others. As he trailed, Mr. Bryce decided to call the left wall the "window wall"; the right wall the "no-window wall"; the wall opposite him the "small-door wall"; and the wall near the entrance the "big-door wall." Remembering the labels would enable Mr. Bryce to orient himself in the future and to ask for help in reaching a destination within the room.

The labeling technique can be applied to any room a person uses. For example, someone in a residential facility can categorize bedroom walls as the "bed wall," the "window wall," the "closet wall," and the "door wall."

After labeling the walls, Mr. Bryce explored the center of the room, which contained many pieces of furniture, using a crisscross pattern of movement. First, he trailed along the right wall to a corner. Then he faced the center of the room and, protecting himself with the upper and lower forearm and hand techniques, crossed to the opposite corner. As he walked along, Mr. Bryce called out the names of the pieces of furniture he passed, a Ping-Pong table and pool table. He repeated the process from two other corners of the room and then returned to the doorway. Now Mr. Bryce could remember the position of the furniture in the room's center relative to the peripheral walls. He had completed the familiarization process.

Lisa repeated that process with Mr. Bryce in other rooms. Within a short time, he was able to find his way around his new home without difficulty.

Another way to aid in familiarization is to tape-record the orientation sessions. Still another way is to use a magnetic board and strips to develop "maps" of the rooms a person is striving to master.

Although teaching them can take some time, familiarization, trailing, and protective techniques save time in the long run because they make people both independent and safe. Ultimately, these skills enhance your programs because they allow people who are visually impaired to participate fully. Everyone benefits when you teach the basics of O&M to those who need to rely on them to get around.

CHAPTER 5

FOCUSING ON READING AND WRITING

Like everyone else, older people generally find reading and writing to be highly enjoyable activities. They know that books keep their minds active and writing keeps them in touch with family members and friends who may live far away.

Unfortunately, when vision loss makes reading and writing more difficult, a person may give up these pleasures, not knowing that there are ways to continue them. Among the resources available for people with visual impairments are large-print books, Talking Books, special writing aids, and low vision aids and devices. Some of these aids are fairly simple, whereas others are "high tech"; the appropriate choice depends on the degree and kind of vision loss. If you familiarize yourself with what is available and learn some simple tips, you can keep the pages turning for someone who would otherwise be cut off from the printed word.

As with other aspects of visual impairment, you need to be alert for evidence of change. You may notice, for example, that an individual who was formerly a strong reader no longer carries a newspaper around or that a person cannot read the instructions for a group activity or has trouble signing his or her name to a document.

First Steps

SHED LIGHT ON THE MATTER

Good lighting is the most basic requirement for reading, writing, and other close work, and sometimes a person's vision problems can be alleviated simply by adjusting the lighting.

But lighting that is comfortable for one person may not be comfortable for another. Some people read and write best in natural light, while others need more light or less light than that. So experiment by closing the curtains or adjusting the blinds on the window in some cases or trying brighter bulbs in others.

If natural light turns out to be sufficient, have the person sit with his or her back to a window. If more light is needed, it should be provided by an incandescent lamp that is directed over the shoulder nearest the person's better eye. Most people find that a 75-watt bulb provides a comfortable level of lighting.

More lighting tips: A gooseneck lamp or high-intensity lamp, directed down onto the area of activity, can increase visibility. A rheostat, which adjusts the level of light in a room, can simplify the search for comfortable lighting. Finally, probably the easiest and most effective thing you can do is to replace burned-out bulbs or remind someone else to do so.

In conjunction with providing better lighting, remembering the importance of contrast is useful. Placing dark-colored objects on light backgrounds, and vice versa, can often help visually impaired people see them. Whether writing black letters on a white sign or putting white cups on a dark tablecloth, this is a key principle to keep in mind.

REFERRAL TO A LOW VISION CENTER

If better lighting does not correct someone's problem, professional help may be required. Advise the person to arrange for an appointment at a low vision center for a diagnostic evaluation or, if appropriate, offer to help him or her make the appointment (see Chapter 1 for more information). Staff at the center specialize in helping people make the most of their remaining vision and often prescribe various reading aids and provide training in their use.

Ways to Facilitate Reading

Among the reading aids that may be prescribed at the low vision center are magnifiers—which can be held in the hand, worn around the neck, mounted on a stand, or attached to eyeglass frames—special filters, or prism lenses. The center will provide training in how to use these devices, but training may also be

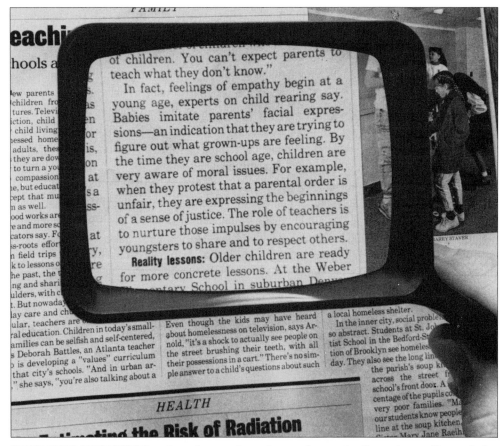

HAND-HELD MAGNIFIERS such as the one shown here enlarge print for easier reading and also offer the convenience of being portable.

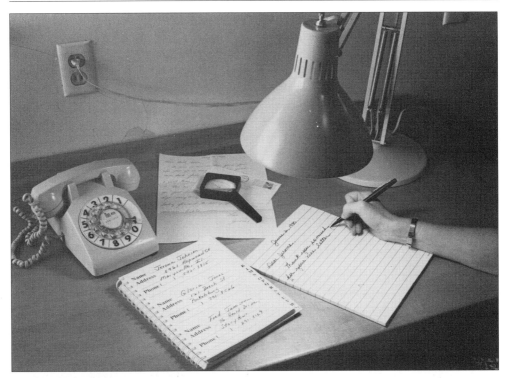

BOLD-LINE PAPER and black felt-tip pens are effective tools for easier writing, especially when used in conjunction with good lighting.

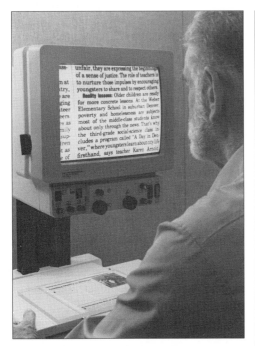

A CLOSED-CIRCUIT TELEVISION projects an enlarged image of a page onto a television screen.

available from state agencies for visually impaired persons or local rehabilitation centers.

There are also high-tech aids on the market that can be useful to facilities serving a significant number of people with serious visual impairments. A closed-circuit television (CCTV) system is an example. It consists of a TV monitor and a platform on which reading material is placed. A camera projects the material onto the monitor in a variety of contrasts and type sizes, making it easier to read.

An optical scanner can also be useful for visually impaired readers. Scanners can be used to translate text into synthetic speech, in a manner similar to the scanners used at the checkout counters of some supermarkets. For information on these and other reading aids, see the Resources section of this book.

LOW VISION DEVICES: USEFUL HINTS

REMIND THE PERSON. A simple question, such as, "Don't you have your magnifier with you, Mr. Reily?" can be a gentle reminder about using the aid or can alert the individual to the fact that he or she forgot to bring it from home or another room in a facility.

BE ENCOURAGING. It takes practice to learn how to use an optical device. At first, reading with an aid may be difficult. Assure the person that this will change. Stress the value of persistence. Supportive comments like, "You're really sticking with it, Mrs. Sanchez," may be helpful.

DISCOURAGE INAPPROPRIATE USE. Since magnifiers and reading glasses can distort depth perception, they are meant for reading and writing only, not for walking around. If you notice someone using a device inappropriately, a tactful reminder may help ensure the person's safety.

LABEL DEVICES. If you work in a residential facility, make sure that aids and eyeglasses are labeled with their owners' names. Labeling prevents not only loss, but the inadvertent use of someone else's aid. It is also important to label other types of aids, such as canes and walkers.

ARRANGE FOR DEMONSTRATIONS. The use of special devices can be the subject of a talk. Good sources of lecturers or demonstrators are the state agency for visually impaired persons, a local agency for visually impaired persons, a low vision center, a company that sells high-tech optical equipment, a library for visually impaired persons, a radio reading service, and the organizations listed in Resources.

TIPS FOR USING LOW VISION DEVICES

If you know that low vision devices have been prescribed for particular individuals, check on their use from time to time. There are several ways to make sure the aids are as valuable as they could be, and these are listed in "Low Vision Devices: Useful Hints."

NONOPTICAL DEVICES TO HELP WITH READING

In addition to low vision devices, there are certain simple items that can facilitate reading:

- A sheet of colored acetate, which can be purchased at most office supply or art supply stores, increases the contrast between type and background when it is put over a page of reading matter.

- A line of print becomes easier to read when a typoscope, a piece of dark plastic or cardboard with a slit in it, is placed over the line, thereby isolating it from the rest of the text. Typoscopes are available from AFB (see Resources).

- The most frequently called numbers in a telephone directory—one of the more difficult publications to read, by the way—can be made more legible by highlighting them with a colored marker. It is also a good idea to make a personal phone book by printing frequently called names and numbers in large print on index cards with a black marker.

- Restaurant menus, theater programs, and other items that are usually read in a dim light can be seen more clearly with the aid of a penlight or pocket-size flashlight.

- A bookstand is not usually thought of as a reading aid, but when a reader's hands are shaky or occupied by a magnifier, it can make the difference between being able to read or giving up. That is why adjustable stands—those that can be set at the correct height and angle for a particular task—are a worthwhile purchase for any center or facility.

LARGE PRINT IS EASY TO FIND

A reading problem can sometimes be solved easily by larger print. Fortunately, large-print books, from best-sellers to reference works, are available at most bookstores and local libraries. A wide variety of other items that have to be read, such as watches, clocks, telephone dials, bathroom scales, playing cards, thermometers, rulers, oven dials, microwave dials, and board games, is also available with large print or in "talking" adaptations that provide information through synthetic speech.

AFB and other organizations and companies that offer these products will gladly send you their catalogs (see Resources). In fact, it is a good idea to have a collection of such catalogs available in a community room for ready browsing.

OTHER WAYS OF READING

"Reading" can also be accomplished without the use of print, through two free services, one on tape and the other on the airwaves.

Talking Books, a program of the National Library Service for the Blind and Physically Handicapped, provides cassettes and disks through the mail (see Resources). Also available are cassette and tape players, an Easy Reader Tape Player with only one button to manipulate, earphones, and remote controls. A person can join the Talking Book program at any local library, which also carries order forms listing the books and magazines that are available. Materials returned to Talking Books may be shipped postage-free if stamped "Free Matter for the Blind." This is also true, incidentally, of all braille letters, large-print letters, or tapes prepared by a visually impaired person.

Radio reading services are provided by radio stations that specialize in the broadcast of printed materials (see Resources). Upon applying to be a subscriber, the individual receives a receiver tuned to the station's frequency and a listing of programs. Most states have at least one such station, and several have more than one, so there's no reason for a person who needs one to be without a radio that "reads."

Ways to Facilitate Writing

Writing skills may diminish at the same time that reading skills do. And, as with reading, there are several steps you can take to make writing less difficult for an older person:

- *Provide contrast*. Without enough contrast between paper and writing surface, the paper's edges can seem to disappear. To create contrast, put a solid-color place mat or a darker piece of paper under the writing paper. Contrast can also be achieved by putting the paper on a clipboard, which has the added advantage of holding the paper steady. Another plus is that the duller surrounding surface provided by the clipboard may help eliminate bothersome glare.
- *Use colored writing paper*. White paper is not the easiest for everyone to see. Experiment with yellow, beige, and gray.
- *Suggest using paper with bold lines*. Adults do not usually use such paper, so a visually impaired person may not realize how much easier it is to keep handwriting straight when following a line. Even if his or her handwriting is shaky or is scarcely legible, encourage the per-

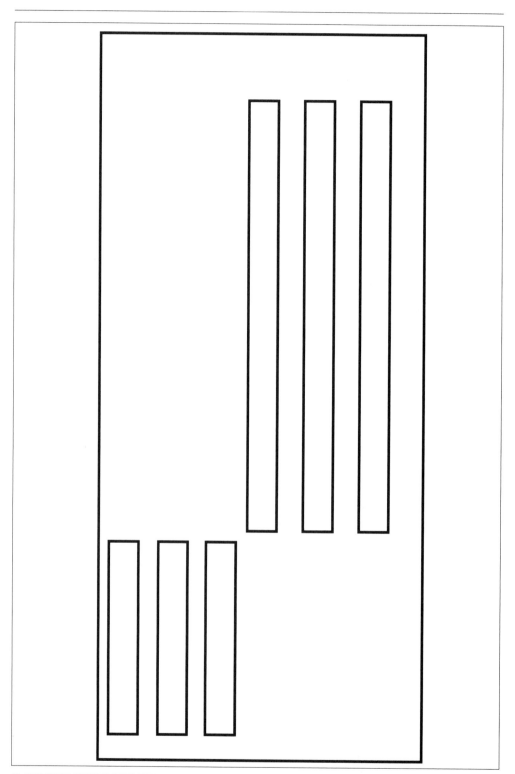

A SAMPLE ENVELOPE-WRITING GUIDE. Envelope guides need to be the standard sizes of envelopes and have cutout lines that correspond with standard "address to" and "address from" areas.

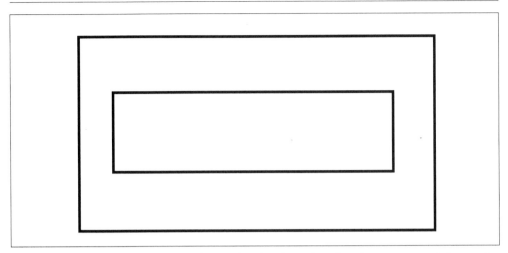

A SAMPLE SIGNATURE GUIDE. Guides can be of various sizes, but the space cut or left open for the signature should be a length that can accommodate the length of the person's name.

son to practice writing, particularly signatures and other combinations of words that are frequently used. If necessary, give the person a supply of lined pads. And suggest that he or she use a pen with a broad felt tip.

• ***Create writing guides***. By demarcating spaces for writing, raised guides made of cardboard or similar material make it easier for the individual to see where to write or feel where to write (if he or she can no longer see the writing). You can use the templates pictured in this chapter to create an envelope-writing guide and a signature guide, thus facilitating the performance of two common writing activities.

In making these guides, it is best to use card stock or poster-board paper, in a dark color, to create contrast with the white or light page on which they are placed. Be sure to provide instruction in using the guides. For example, you can paper clip a signature guide on a sheet of paper, turn it to the angle at which the person usually writes, and watch while he or she practices a few times. Ready-made guides are also available from many of the organizations listed in Resources.

• ***Make your own communications clear***. When writing to a visually impaired person, remember that print made by a typewriter or word processor is the easiest to read. Use large-size characters. If you must write by hand, use mainly lower-case letters instead of all capitals, which are more difficult to decipher. Use a pen with a broad felt tip and dark color ink.

If a visually impaired person has typewriting skills, encourage him or her to keep using them. Stress the fact that, as with other types of writing, spelling mistakes and crossed-out words do not matter. What is important is to keep up communication with those we care about.

Another way to communicate, if one finds writing difficult, is to send "letters" recorded on tape cassettes. Because they are so convenient, tape recorders should be available in every facility, just as are pencils, pens, and paper. Try to make certain that you have tape recorders on hand. Show people how they work. Encourage those who have stopped writing to make tapes for friends and loved ones, perhaps on a weekly basis. Tapes bridge the miles and any generation gap, since children enjoy listening to them as much as older people enjoy making them.

With all the resources available, no one has to be without the ability to read or write, in one form or another. By keeping tabs on the abilities of the people you work with and being familiar with ways of helping them, you can make certain that they continue to enjoy the pleasure of words for many years to come.

CHAPTER 6

TECHNIQUES FOR MEALTIME

Eating is a necessity, but it can be a lot more than that. Eating is a social activity as well, and an opportunity to get together with friends.

But meals can also be a source of embarrassment if one has difficulty finding food and utensils. Even a slight vision loss—the type of loss experienced by most older people with vision problems—can make mealtimes more difficult.

A dining table is usually crowded with items. Just think about all the objects you ordinarily see. Now imagine that you are seeing them a little less clearly. Would you be able to tell the salt shaker from the pepper shaker? The water pitcher from the coffee server? This is the type of difficulty that can cause accidents—and a retreat from the dining room.

After he spilled the water pitcher several meals in a row, Mr. Cohen told Eva Rossi, the recreational counselor at the life-care community where he lived, that he would eat in his apartment from then on instead of in the community dining room. Eva realized how unpleasant it would be for Mr. Cohen to be cut off from his friends. She also knew that his vision loss was not particularly severe. He could easily see his plate, knife, and fork, but he had difficulty identifying items that were less familiar or farther away. So Eva asked Mr. Cohen if he would agree to have her assist him for a while.

For the next few days, Eva sat next to Mr. Cohen at meals, pointing out the location of the serving dishes, the water pitcher, the salad bowl, and so forth. With just this bit of help, Mr. Cohen was able to ask for what he wanted or to reach for it without causing a spill. And, as soon as the other diners understood the problem, they were able to take over the helping role. Of equal importance, Mr. Cohen learned how to assert himself and ask for the information he needed.

Most older people with vision problems need only a little assistance from others, plus awareness that they can benefit from verbal clues. However, the relatively small number of people with more severe visual impairments need to learn special techniques to feed themselves independently. There are techniques for locating the place setting, remembering where foods are on the plate, using a knife to spread or cut, pouring liquids, and adding seasonings to food.

Although teaching such techniques may sound formidable, this is really not the case, once you have become familiar with them. Reading about the techniques here and perhaps practicing them a bit should give you all the preparation you need.

When you teach these skills, though, remember two important rules. First, make sure the person wants your help. Even an individual with significant vision loss may prefer to do things, or not do them, by his or her own "method."

Second, make sure the teaching takes place in private. Find a quiet room with a table and set up a place setting and accompanying serving dishes for a practice session. Or, depending on the circumstances, such as in a center or residential environment, perhaps you can ask the kitchen staff to put one place setting, some serving dishes with food, and a pitcher on a table when the dining room is empty, so you can work with the person alone. If possible, put the plate on a mat of contrasting color, which will make it more visible.

Eva Rossi arranged for such a setup when she started to work with Mrs. Lucas, a resident whose vision loss was more severe than Mr. Cohen's. By following the procedures Eva used with Mrs. Lucas, you can learn how to teach eating skills.

Getting Settled at the Table

First, Eva made sure that the table was positioned so Mrs. Lucas could travel to it easily and well lit so she could see the place setting. Then Eva had Mrs. Lucas stand behind a chair. She placed Mrs. Lucas's hand on the back and told her to pull the chair away from the table. Eva asked Mrs. Lucas to run her hand over the seat to see if there was anything lying on it. After making sure the chair was clear of objects, Mrs. Lucas moved to the front of it, sat down, and pulled herself in. She made certain her body was perpendicular to the table by lightly running the backs of her hands along the table's edge.

Mrs. Lucas could easily feel where the plate and the utensils were. To find the other items at her setting, Eva told Mrs. Lucas to trail gently along the table, keeping her fingers on the surface at all times to avoid knocking things over. (The position of the hand in trailing is shown in Chapter 4.)

The first objective was to locate the coffee cup and commit its location to memory. With the back of her fingers, Mrs. Lucas found the cup and grasped it with her right hand, her dominant hand. As she lifted the cup, Mrs. Lucas put her left hand where the cup had been and made a mental note of the spot. This allowed her to put the cup back in the same place.

Mrs. Lucas repeated the locating procedure to find the water glass and the water pitcher. She was then ready to eat her meal. Eva reminded Mrs. Lucas to lean forward slightly over the table. By doing so, her face would be positioned over the plate and her hands would be close to the plate.

Dining around the Clock

Mrs. Lucas's plate contained peas, mashed potatoes, and ham steak. How could Mrs. Lucas learn the location of these foods without touching them with her fingers?

Eva asked Mrs. Lucas to think of the plate as a clock. "Your peas are at 12 o'clock," she said, "the mashed potatoes at 3 o'clock, and the ham steak at 6 o'clock." Of course, Eva made certain to turn the plate so the foods were actually at the "times" she announced.

With the clock image in mind, it was easy for Mrs. Lucas to remember where the foods were. She also realized that by asking a dining companion to use this technique, she could locate the foods on her plate at any meal. In addition, the clock technique could be used to tell her where a glass, a bread plate, or other items near the plate were located.

A Spreading and Cutting Edge

Eating requires more maneuvering of objects than we usually realize. Spreading butter, for example, takes no thought when one can easily see the butter, the bread, and the knife, but if a person has visual difficulties, a special technique is needed.

Eva told Mrs. Lucas that the first step was to "explore" the butter with her knife, that is, run it gently over the top of the butter to find out how much there was and how much she needed. Next, Eva had Mrs. Lucas cut off some butter; place it in the center of the bread; and spread it out from the center to the edges, which Mrs. Lucas could feel with her fingers.

Eva explained that the same technique, moving from the middle out to the edges, could be used for spreading jelly, mustard, mayonnaise, and any other "spread." The back of a spoon would work just as well as a knife.

To learn how to cut meat—a more difficult task than spreading butter—Eva had Mrs. Lucas first identify the cutting edge of the knife with her fingers, then locate the edge of the ham steak with her knife and keep the knife there. Mrs. Lucas put her fork into the steak about a half inch from the edge. Starting at the edge, Mrs. Lucas cut a semicircle around the fork with the knife. She held the steak down with the knife while she lifted the fork to eat the piece of ham. Then she put the fork back into the steak near the knife and cut the next piece in the same fashion. The idea was to keep the steak under her control at all times.

Mrs. Lucas succeeded in cutting the ham steak, but some people with vision loss have difficulty; the meat may be tough and the semicircle process is slow going. Often, it is simpler to ask for help in cutting meat. If the cutting can be done in the kitchen before the food comes to the table, so much the better for a person's sense of self-esteem.

Eva taught Mrs. Lucas one other eating tip: Use a "pusher," a piece of roll or bread, to push items like peas together, so they can be scooped up easily with a fork. If bread is not available, a spoon can serve the same purpose.

From Pitcher to Cup

The practice meal Eva arranged included a pitcher of water so Mrs. Lucas could learn how to pour cold liquids. First, Eva had Mrs. Lucas trail along the table with her right hand—her dominant hand, remember—to locate the pitcher. Mrs. Lucas ran her hand up the pitcher, found the spout, and turned the pitcher so the spout was facing her cup. Then she wrapped the middle finger and thumb of her left hand around the cup and placed her index finger across the top.

Mrs. Lucas brought the cup up toward the pitcher, lining up her index finger with the spout. Keeping the cup raised and lifting the pitcher slightly, she poured until she could feel the water reach her finger. Then Mrs. Lucas put down the pitcher and the cup and readjusted her fingers so she could drink comfortably.

Attempts to use the same technique with hot liquids need to be modified to avoid the possibility of scalding. It is helpful to move slowly and to pay particular attention to the proximity of the heat emanating from the liquid. Fingers should not be placed in the path of hot liquids. Therefore, for such liquids, Eva explained, Mrs. Lucas could use an indicator that beeps when the coffee gets near the top of the cup. Indicators of this kind are available from AFB and other organizations that provide adaptive equipment (see Resources). Another way for a person to judge the height of liquid is to put a small object in the bottom of the cup and to pour until he or she can feel that it has floated to the top.

Adding Salt and Pepper

Eva observed that Mrs. Lucas poured too much salt on her food because she had difficulty judging how much she was pouring. So Eva showed Mrs. Lucas this simple way to estimate the right amount of salt or pepper: Pour a small amount into the palm of one hand. Take a pinch with the other hand and sprinkle it over the food. Taste the food, and if you have not sprinkled enough, add a bit more. Remember to add seasoning bit by bit. You can always put on more salt or pepper, but you cannot take it away.

After her practice meal, Mrs. Lucas felt much more confident about her ability to dine on her own and was eager to try it. Eva reminded her, though, not to be afraid to ask for help if she needed it; that is what friends, including staff and volunteers, are for. Using occasional assistance does not mean that one's independence has been compromised. A little flexibility can go a long way, Eva advised, toward making mealtimes more comfortable for everyone.

And the skills that Eva taught Mrs. Lucas can make mealtimes more comfortable, too. The skills are not difficult to learn, and since most visually impaired people are highly motivated, the skills are not really difficult to teach either. Every time you take the time to learn and to teach, you improve the quality of a person's life when it might otherwise have been diminished. In short, you share the bounties of life's table with those around you.

CHAPTER 7

TIME, MONEY, AND OTHER ESSENTIALS

The majority of older people who are visually impaired have no trouble exchanging money, figuring out what time it is, or making a telephone call. But others need a system for doing these tasks or special assistance in the form of adaptive equipment.

Just imagine what it would be like not to be able to tell one coin from another by sight or to check out the time simply by glancing at the clock. Frustrating? Well, you can help end that frustration by demonstrating some alternative ways of getting these things done.

Money

Begin with something that is basic to independence and to everyday life: money. Coins can be identified by the way they feel, and bills can be folded in ways that make them identifiable. Here's how you can teach these easy-to-follow methods.

IDENTIFYING COINS BY TOUCH

One at a time, put a penny, a nickel, a dime, a quarter, and a half-dollar in the hand of the person with whom you are working. Then have the person finger the coins. Ask him or her to observe the following:

- *Size*. The dime is the smallest coin, and the half-dollar is the largest.

- *Edge*. The penny and the nickel have smooth edges. The dime, the quarter, and the half-dollar have milled, rough edges.
- *Thickness*. The nickel is thicker than the other coins.

Have the person practice identifying the various coins. A nickel is fairly easy to recognize because of its thickness, and the dime, because of its size. The penny is the only coin of usual thickness to have a smooth edge. A coin that is larger than a dime and has a milled edge has to be a quarter or half-dollar.

The more time one spends feeling the coins, the easier it is to remember the differences and to become expert at identification.

IDENTIFYING BILLS BY THEIR FOLD

By folding denominations of bills in different ways, a visually impaired person can easily locate them in a wallet. The most commonly used method is outlined in "How to Identify Money by Fold."

Encourage the person you are helping to experiment with ways of carrying bills. For example, some people find it easier to have bills of only one or two denominations in their wallets.

To have the person you are helping practice identifying money, fold some bills and put them in an envelope with several coins. Ask him or her to open the envelope and tell you what is inside.

Another technique is to have the individual fold some bills and put them in a wallet. Then pretend you are in a grocery store and have him or her purchase something from you—a carton of milk, for example. Give both bills and coins as change and ask the person to identify them. Remind the person that in an actual shopping situation, it can sometimes be a good idea to ask for a verbal recitation of the change.

Eyes or Fingers on the Time

Most visually impaired people can see a clock or watch if the numbers are large enough, and a woman need not hesitate to use a man's watch if that's the only kind she can find with such numbers. The watch selected should have a simple face, with black numbers on a white background or another effective contrast. Roman numerals, which are difficult to read, should be avoided.

Another option, if a suitable timepiece cannot be found in a store, is to purchase a large-number watch or talking watch. AFB and other organizations sell these

watches and other products made especially for people with visual impairments (see Resources).

If the person you are working with has a significant visual impairment, a braille watch, with which the wearer relies on the sense of touch to tell time, may be a good choice. Remember, though, that sensation in the person's hands and fingers must be unimpaired to use such a watch.

Braille is a system of writing for people with visual impairments that uses characters made up of raised dots. On a braille watch, the raised dots are placed near the regular numbers in this fashion:

- *12:00:* three dots arranged vertically
- *3:00 and 9:00:* two dots arranged horizontally
- *6:00:* two dots arranged vertically
- *Other hours:* one dot.

A person tells the time by feeling the direction of the large and small hands and the dots. If your facility or center serves a number of visually impaired people, it may want to purchase a braille watch for demonstration purposes. That way, you can sit down with someone, review the positioning of the dots on the watch, and allow time for practice.

Braille watches and clocks with large numbers are available from AFB and other organizations that distribute adaptive equipment. Also available is a variety of other items that talk or have large numbers: bathroom scales, playing cards, thermometers, rulers, microwave dials, games, and telephone templates (see Resources).

Making Phones Easy to Use

The numbers on telephones are easier to read when they are in large print. A variety of easy-to-read numbers on telephone templates that have adhesive backings and can be placed on telephones is available. These templates are made for both Touch-tone and rotary phones, and information about them can be obtained from AFB and other organizations in Resources.

In addition to the templates, you should also know about these two methods of teaching people to use the telephone by feel:

- **For Touch-tone phones**. Have the person run his or her dominant hand—the one used for dialing—from left to right over the second horizontal row of the telephone pad and place the middle three fingers on 4, 5, and 6. With the fingers thus positioned, it is easy to remember that 1, 2, and 3 are located just above and 7, 8, and 9 just below. The middle finger can be used to press zero, which is located just below 8.
- **For dial or rotary phones**. Have the person memorize the numbers and letters represented by the holes. To dial, he or she should place the first four fingers in the first four holes, with the little finger in 1, ring finger in 2, middle finger in 3, and index finger in 4. The index finger is moved to dial the numbers 5, 6, 7, 8, 9, and zero.

Also bear in mind that there are many models of telephones on the market today for people who are visually impaired. Among the features available are large-print numbers, memory for frequently called telephone numbers, and video screens.

With time and patience, the person you are helping can learn to perform those "small" tasks that mean so much to independence: using the telephone, telling the time, and identifying money. And you can have the satisfaction of knowing that your assistance will be remembered every time the person goes to a store, looks at a watch, or picks up the phone.

CHAPTER 8

TOWARD BETTER HOUSEKEEPING AND PERSONAL CARE

Taking care of oneself and taking care of one's living quarters go together, and they are the cornerstones of independence. No matter where an older person or anyone else lives—in an apartment, a retirement community, a residential facility, or a private house—housekeeping turns a mere place into a home. And there really is no place like home when it comes to the way we think about ourselves. If we cannot feel capable at home, we are not likely to feel capable anywhere else.

Most older people with vision loss can continue to care for their living quarters and themselves. These activities of daily living (ADLs) can be done more successfully, however, by organizing for both ease and safety. Many older people, for example, do not have enough light in their homes to be safe. That is one of the things that should be changed by proper reorganization.

If you work in a residential setting, you may play a role in teaching personal care techniques or helping a person rearrange his or her quarters. But even if you are not likely to visit the homes of the people you work with, you can still discuss ways to increase safety and efficiency.

Making Living Quarters More Livable

Here is some basic advice that you can give people about making their environment safe and well organized. It is founded on four important principles—increase lighting, eliminate hazards, create color contrast, and organize and label items.

INCREASE LIGHTING

- Use stronger light bulbs or three-way bulbs to provide nonglare lighting.
- Put lamps in places where you do close work; for example, put a gooseneck lamp in the reading-writing area.
- Install extra lights in the bedroom closet and other frequently used closets in other rooms.
- Put special lighting over all stairways, the places where accidents are most likely to occur.
- Make sure that the lighting level is consistent throughout the house so shadows and dangerous bright spots are eliminated. Install rheostats.
- Be certain you can easily reach light switches from doorways and from your bed.
- Use a night-light in the bedroom and in the hallway.

ELIMINATE HAZARDS

- To prevent missing your front door, mark it with a brightly colored Welcome sign.
- Mark thermostats with HiMarks, a highly tactile, sticky substance in a fluorescent orange color, available from AFB (see Resources).
- Replace worn carpeting and floor covering.
- Tape down rugs and electrical cords.
- Use nonskid, nonglare wax to polish floors.
- Close closet doors, drawers, and cupboards as soon as you have taken out needed objects.
- Keep desk chairs and table chairs pushed in.
- Move large pieces of furniture out of the main traffic area. Or cover the edges with a brightly colored pad or a towel of a contrasting color.
- Pick up shoes, clothing, books, and other items that you could trip over. In fact, put an object away when you are through using it, for safety's sake and so you can easily find it again.
- Mop up spills as soon as they occur.

CREATE COLOR CONTRAST

- Place light objects against a dark background, a white table near a green wall or a black switchplate on a white wall.
- Install doorknobs that contrast in color with the door.
- Avoid upholstery with patterns. Stripes and checks create confusion, rather than contrast.

ORGANIZE AND LABEL ITEMS

- Keep items that are used together near each other—on the same shelf, in the same closet, or in the same box.
- Label each box with a black felt-tip pen. Or write the contents on index cards and wrap the cards around the boxes with rubber bands. Self-adhesive labels can also be used.
- Create labels with the Voxcom Card Recorder Kit, available from AFB, if you have severe vision loss. As you speak into a cassette recorder, it produces self-adhering strips of magnetic recording tape.

Although these four major principles apply to every portion of someone's living space, some rooms or areas require special consideration. Certain housekeeping problems may arise in specific rooms, but there are uncomplicated ways in which they can be handled.

Tips for Various Rooms

THE KITCHEN:
"I DON'T KNOW WHICH CAN I'M OPENING"

Mr. Goodman mentioned to Robert, a counselor at a community center he attended regularly, that he had eaten only corn the night before. "I opened three cans that I thought were corn, salmon, and pineapple," he said, but "each one turned out to be corn." Mr. Goodman laughed, but it was obvious that he was annoyed at himself.

Robert told Mr. Goodman that it is important to label cans as soon as they come into the house. They can be marked with felt stick-ons, self-adhesive labels, or index cards bearing large letters, such as "PEP" for pepper or "CIN" for cinnamon. Another method is to use varying numbers of rubber bands for identification: one band for one type of product, two bands for another, and so forth.

Robert also told Mr. Goodman to label all other cooking supplies. He advised that staples, such as spices, salt, and sugar, be transferred to wide-mouth containers. By bending a metal measuring spoon to a 90-

degree angle, Mr. Goodman could scoop out ingredients easily.

To identify settings on the oven dial, Robert suggested using dabs of HiMarks, which can be molded into peaks and easily felt. Robert also suggested attaching lights to the underside of the cabinets over the counter and gluing light and dark squares of plastic to the counter itself. The latter would allow Mr. Goodman to work with dark ingredients on the light-colored squares and light ingredients on the dark squares. When slicing food, he could use a cutting board of contrasting color, thus making the food more visible.

Robert also gave Mr. Goodman some additional dos and don'ts to observe in the kitchen, which are listed in "Hints for the Kitchen." Mr. Goodman found many of Robert's suggestions useful. By following them, he found that he was able to produce meals he could both identify and enjoy.

HINTS FOR THE KITCHEN

DON'T
- Store spices above the stove.
- Remove a pan from the stove before you turn off the flame.
- Wear loose clothing when cooking.

DO
- Wear short sleeves or tapered sleeves.
- Put splatter screens under pans.
- Use oven mitts to handle pans.
- Set a timer to remind you when to turn off the stove or other electrical appliances.
- Maintain all appliances in good condition. Don't overload circuits.
- Use knife-cutting guides, available from AFB, to cut meats and other foods.

THE BEDROOM: "I CAN'T FIND THE CLOTHES I WANT"

Mrs. Moran's bureau drawers were always overflowing, crammed with underwear, blouses, and sweaters. Until she experienced some vision loss, Mrs. Moran had no difficulty putting an outfit together, but nowadays she always looked slightly disheveled.

Jennifer, an aide who worked in the residential facility where Mrs. Moran lived, was able to help her organize more successfully. First, with Jennifer's assistance, Mrs. Moran decided which clothing to give away. Then she reorganized her bureau and closet according to the following guidelines:

- *Divide and conquer*. Mrs. Moran placed dividers in her drawers to keep items separate and easily visible.
- *Organize by outfit*. Mrs. Moran put the components of each major outfit—a blouse, skirt, and jacket, for example—together. She hung some outfits in the closet and folded others together in a bureau drawer. Another way Mrs. Moran could have organized is to keep all clothing of the same color together. That way, it is easy to find items that match or complement each other.
- *Label with safety pins*. Mrs. Moran put a single pin on the components of one outfit, two pins on the components of another one, and so forth. If she had organized by color, she could have placed safety pins in one direction for red clothing, in another direction for green clothing, and used various combinations for other colors. Other ways of labeling are to use French knots, colored tape, colored stickers, or braille tags.
- *Bag it*. Mrs. Moran put small, easily lost items, such as jewelry, in plastic bags. She bagged scarves and belts that went with an outfit together and hung each

bag in the closet near the appropriate outfit.

- *Label and organize makeup*. Mrs. Moran labeled all her cosmetics and put them in a large basket. She placed the basket near the illuminated magnifying mirror that Jennifer suggested she use to put on makeup. Jennifer also told Mrs. Moran that makeup could be applied more easily if she selected light-colored foundation and lipstick. She showed Mrs. Moran how to apply the lipstick in dabs, working from the corners of the mouth to the middle.

Finally, Jennifer told Mrs. Moran to be sure to examine clothing regularly in a good light for spots and rips and to take care of repairs at once.

By maintaining her wardrobe in good condition and organizing it efficiently, Mrs. Moran found that she was able to reclaim the well-dressed look she prized.

THE BATHROOM: "I'M AFRAID OF FALLING, AGAIN"

Even a slight degree of vision loss can make the bathroom—with its tile and slippery surfaces—a scary place. After Mr. Romero fell in the bathroom, he felt uncomfortable there, so he asked Carole, an administrative assistant at the retirement community where he lived, for some help.

Carole looked over the bathroom and gave Mr. Romero these tips, based on the four concepts of increasing lighting, eliminating hazards, using color contrast, and labeling items:

- Make sure that all rugs in the bath area are nonskid.
- Keep frequently used items in the same place at all times. Label them. Whenever possible, choose plastic, rather than glass, containers.
- Buy towels, washcloths, and bath mats that contrast in color with the tub and tile.
- Use hand soaps and shampoos in pump dispensers to prevent spillage. Buy bar soaps in bright colors that can be easily seen.
- Put a nonskid mat, friction tape, or patterned appliques on the bottom of the tub or the floor of the shower. Select colors that contrast with the surface.
- Hang a shower caddy in the shower to hold soap and shampoo.
- Install a grab bar on the edge of the tub or a railing on the wall of the shower to help prevent slipping when getting in and out.
- Install additional lighting—it should be impervious to dampness—over the tub and shower.
- Replace a white toilet seat with a darker, contrasting seat. If necessary, put a frame with arms over the seat for ease of seating.

Like many older people, Mr. Romero had specific questions about how to bathe himself and perform other personal care tasks. Here are the questions he asked Carole, along with the answers she gave him:

- *How can I wash without scalding myself?* Learn how far you have to rotate faucets to get the temperature you want. Turn on the cold water first, then add the hot; turn off the hot water first, then the cold. In the shower, use a handheld shower so you can test the water temperature on your hand.
- *How can I tell how much water is in the tub?* Sit on the edge of the tub, or kneel or squat beside it, and put your hand in the water. To judge visually, there are several methods: Put a contrasting strip of tape at the desired height, drape a towel over the tub and turn off the water when the edge becomes wet, or use a water-level indicator.
- *How can I get the right amount of toothpaste on the brush?* Use a dark

color or striped toothpaste. Hold the bristles of the brush between your thumb and forefinger. That way, you will be able to judge the amount of toothpaste as you squeeze it from the tube. Another method is to squeeze the toothpaste directly into your mouth. When you use tooth powder, shake the powder into a cup and dunk the brush into it.

- *Should I cut my nails or file them?* Filing is safer than using a scissors or a clipper. If you have diabetes, be certain that only a medical professional cuts your toenails.
- *Should I shave with a regular shaver or an electric one?* Use an electric shaver. It is less likely to cause nicks and cuts.
- *How can I tell my medicines apart?* If possible, keep the medications in alphabetical order. If you cannot identify a medication bottle by its size, shape, or color, label it in large type or print. Or use strips of adhesive in vertical, horizontal, or diagonal patterns.

Mr. Romero found Carole's answers useful and reassuring. By making his bathroom safer, he was able to overcome his fear of falling and perform personal care tasks more efficiently.

Basic Housekeeping Activities

There are many tasks to be done around a house, as we all know, and a visually impaired person can accomplish them as well as the rest of us. But special know-how can make some common chores simpler to perform. If you know someone who is struggling with dusting, sweeping, and other jobs, here are some suggestions:

- *Dusting.* Keep all cleaning supplies in a bucket or plastic bin. Dust in an organized pattern. Concentrate on one area of the room at a time. Spray polish directly onto the rag, not on the surface of the furniture. To dust small objects, use a feather duster.
- *Sweeping.* Sweep one small section at a time. After using the dustpan, pick up any leftover dust with a damp paper towel.
- *Laundry.* Put a lamp near the washing machine. Mark key dial settings with HiMarks, glue, or puff paint (the type of paint commonly used to decorate T-shirts). Use safety pins or clip-type clothespins to keep socks together or tuck the socks together.
- *Ironing.* Use a raised ironing board, if the position is not too tiring for your arm. Select a solid-color ironing board cover, rather than one with a pattern. Mark the key settings on the iron. Use a funnel to pour water into a steam iron. Sit down while you iron. To find out if wrinkles have been removed, run your hand over the ironed part of a garment.
- *Mending.* Use a metal-loop needle threader or self-threading needles, available in any notions store. Or stick a needle in a bar of soap while threading it, so both your hands are free. Place the fabric you are sewing on a contrasting surface. Keep a magnet nearby to pick up dropped needles and pins.

When to Keep Hands Off

If you work in a retirement community, life-care center, or other place in which people live, there are a few special principles to remember. The first is that a resident's living space is his or her own. Though you can offer suggestions, it is far better not to try to impose your view of how things should be organized. Some people are upset by changes or embarrassed by too many adaptations. Or they have their own ideas about what they want. As much as possible, always respect an individual's wishes.

Second, never move furniture and personal items, especially medications, without the owner's knowledge and assistance. Not only is it disrespectful to do so, it is dangerous. If you clean an area, make sure that objects are put back where they belong. With caring and courtesy, you can help a visually impaired person turn any type of living quarters into a place in which to be comfortable—a true home.

CHAPTER 9

A SAFE ENVIRONMENT

We have talked about promoting safety and efficiency in an older person's living space. But what about other environments where that person spends a great deal of time? Are they equally safe? Whether you work in a community center, senior citizens' center, residential facility, or nursing home, you can answer this question by taking a good look around.

The factors that help make an environment safe for visually impaired people have already been outlined in Chapter 8 in regard to the home: sufficient lighting, the elimination of hazards, the use of color contrast, and the use of organization and labeling. When these principles are observed, people with vision problems feel comfortable; they also perform activities more efficiently and participate more actively in programs. The result is that everything runs more smoothly, and the environment becomes safer for everyone.

Basic Factors

Here are guidelines for an environment that protects all older people—both those who are visually impaired and others. As you read them, think about how your environment stacks up.

LIGHTING

Lighting should be adapted to the purpose of the room. Hallways, for example, can be well lit by fluorescent lighting. In common rooms and areas where reading, crafts, board games, and other activities are pursued, incandescent lighting should be provided by floor lamps and table lamps. Light should always be aimed at the task at hand, not at the eyes. Mirrors should be placed so the lighting does not reflect off them and create glare. Adjustable blinds, sheer curtains, or draperies are good choices for windows because they allow for the adjustment of natural light. All blinds and draperies should be in working order, and old light bulbs should be replaced regularly.

COLOR CONTRAST

Dark furniture should be placed on light rugs, and vice versa. Walls and carpets should be of contrasting colors, and door frames and handrails should contrast with the wall. Wallpaper in a light pattern can make a dark door easier to see, particularly if a room has several doors. The edges of all steps and ramps should be marked by a contrasting color. Furniture should be selected for texture as well as color, since texture provides tactile clues to identification.

FURNITURE ARRANGEMENT

In recreation rooms and lounges, furniture should be arranged in small groupings so people can converse easily. Accessories in bright colors can make a furniture grouping easier to find. Lamps should be placed to the side of the groupings or behind them. It is a good idea to put some individual chairs near windows for reading in natural light.

FLOOR COVERINGS

Elaborate patterns, which can be confusing, should be avoided. Carpeting should be inspected regularly for tears and wrinkles that can cause falls. Bare floors should be waxed with nonskid, nonglare wax to reduce glare and prevent skids.

SIGNS

Signs throughout should be at eye level, with lettering in a contrasting color. Notices on bulletin boards and walls should be in large print. If a number of people using a building have significant vision problems, braille and raised letters should be on strategic signs. (For more information about signs that are helpful for visually impaired persons and useful in meeting federal requirements, see *Strategies for Community Access: Braille and Raised Large-Print Facility Signs*, a videotape available from AFB.)

STRUCTURAL FEATURES

Revolving doors should have conventional doors on either side of them. Glass doors should be well marked. Door handles and knobs should be standard throughout the facility so they are easily recognizable. Telephone booths, drinking fountains, and fire extinguishers should be recessed in the walls. Railings should extend beyond the top and bottom steps, and landings should be clearly marked. Braille or large numbers in raised lettering should be used

in elevators. Emergency signals should always be both visible and audible.

A Tour with Pen in Hand

The best way to find out what is going on in your center or facility is to take a walk around, starting at the entrance. Your objective is to find out—and list—whatever barriers you may discover to safety and independence. You may want to take along several other employees or volunteers and perhaps some clients as well. It is also a good idea to consult with a professional who understands the accommodations required for disabled persons by the recently implemented Americans with Disabilities Act (ADA) (see Chapter 12; more information is also available from AFB).

As you walk around, observe lighting, color contrast, and the placement of furniture. Does furniture stick out into areas of traffic? Are there torn pieces of carpeting or slippery floors? These questions are just for starters. Others you can think about as you move from place to place are listed in "A Checklist for Safety and Access."

If You Find That Changes Are Needed

It would be the perfect environment that has no problems, so your tour will probably uncover at least a few things that should be changed. When you finish walking around, look over your checklist. Group your discoveries according to category—lighting, color contrast, furniture arrangement, floor coverings, signs, and structural features. Then set to work identifying solutions. Refer to the guidelines offered at the start of this chapter to get an idea of how things should be. If you toured the building with a group, brainstorm with its members. Many heads—like many eyes—are better than one.

A CHECKLIST FOR SAFETY AND ACCESS

THE ENTRANCE

☐ Are the curb and outside steps marked with a contrasting color?

☐ Are glass doors marked to make them more visible?

☐ If there is a revolving door, are there conventional doors on either side?

☐ Does the wheelchair ramp have a nonslip surface?

PUBLIC TELEPHONE AREA

☐ Is the area accessible from the most commonly used rooms?

☐ Do telephone booths protrude into traffic areas?

☐ Do some of the telephones have large-print dials?

☐ Are telephone amplifiers, which increase the level of sound, available?

MAILBOX AREA

☐ Is the area brightly lit?

☐ Are the names and numbers easy to read?

☐ Are the boxes that belong to visually impaired people identified with a bright dot or a label?

HALLWAYS

☐ Is lighting uniform throughout, or are some areas light and others dark?

☐ Are drinking fountains and fire extinguishers located along one wall only and recessed?

☐ Is equipment lying around in the halls?

☐ Are ramps identifiable by a tactile change in surface?

☐ Are emergency exits clearly marked?

STAIRWAYS AND ELEVATORS

☐ Are stairwells clearly lit?

☐ Are landings marked in a contrasting color?

☐ Are the Up and Down lights of elevators easy to see?

☐ Can floor buttons in elevators be identified by both sight and touch?

☐ Are floors also identified by an audible signal?

RECREATION ROOMS, DINING ROOMS, AND OTHER COMMON ROOMS

☐ Are there multiple sources of light?

☐ Does natural light come through?

☐ Do furniture, carpeting, and walls contrast with each other?

☐ Is there furniture obstructing areas of traffic?

☐ Are dining room chairs pushed in under the tables?

☐ Are rooms soundproofed so that conversation can be carried on easily?

COMMON BATHROOMS

☐ Are the signs identifying the men's room and the women's room large enough to read and easy to feel?

☐ Do fixtures contrast in color with walls and floors?

☐ Are there grab bars along the wall, on the bathtub, and in the shower?

☐ Are the cold- and hot-water faucets clearly marked?

☐ Are rugs and bath mats nonskid?

- Establish priorities among the solutions for each category, giving the highest priority to the most hazardous situations and to those that are most economical. For example, it is fairly inexpensive to put nonskid, nonglare wax on floors; increase the amount of light in a room; get blinds in working order; or mark the landing of a stairwell with colored paint. It may be more expensive to create contrast by painting walls, floors, and doors and even more costly to convert elevators so that a sound signals the floors. Modifications in the structure of the building itself are likely to be the most costly.
- Create a "wish list" of environmental modifications, and meet with your administrator to discuss the list. If other people are working with you, they should attend the meeting, too. Your list should include the two most important solutions for each category.
- In talking with your administrator, point out that a safer environment benefits not only visually impaired people but everyone else as well. Many modifications may also be required by the ADA. If your administrator is not familiar with the guidelines offered in this chapter, you may want to review some of them with him or her.
- Extensive modifications, such as changes in the building structure, may require approval from the board of directors or other governing or executive body of a center or facility. If you and your administrator suggest modifications, be sure to have an idea of the costs involved and what the time frame will be for making the changes. You should also present a plan that includes short-term and long-term goals.
- Fortunately, several types of professionals, such as rehabilitation specialists and architects, can help you with planning.

You can also refer to a document that reviews safety considerations: *American National Standards for Providing Accessibility and Usability for Physically Handicapped People,* produced by the American National Standards Institute. A consultant from AFB can tell you how to meet the institute's requirements.

If agreement is reached about undertaking major modifications, they may still have to wait until funding sources are found for work to begin. As work proceeds, you can encourage everyone by posting photographs of each modification as it is begun and completed. Be sure to congratulate yourself, too, for having taken a stand on behalf of a better environment.

Keeping a Personal Eye on Safety

While any modifications are in progress, remember to do all you can to promote safety in the meantime. If you spot hazards, such as torn rugs, damp floors, or holes in sidewalks, tell people with visual problems to avoid them. Also report all hazards to housekeeping or janitorial staff, and check back to make certain that they get fixed. In addition, the following four points are vital:

1. Offer people help in situations where they may hurt themselves, such as going from outdoors to indoors or traveling a corridor with wet floors.
2. Review the building's safety features with visually impaired people. Show them where the fire alarms and emergency stairs are located. Then have them show you that they can find the alarm and the stairs by counting the doors along a corridor or by counting the number of steps they have to take. Demonstrate how to turn on the alarm and how to open the windows to fire escapes.

3. Ask your administrator to go over fire-drill procedures with you. During an actual drill, observe what happens. Are the people who would need vision aids or walkers in an actual emergency using them now? They should be. And they should be given enough time to practice evacuation procedures to feel comfortable with them.

4. Advise all the people you work with to report suspicious odors or smoke immediately—and to investigate afterward. Advise people, too, never to smoke in bed and to dispose of cigarettes safely. By observing these precautions, they may never have to take part in an actual evacuation.

By keeping all aspects of safety uppermost in your mind, you can make a big difference in the environment of that important place where you work with—and help—older people.

CHAPTER 10

A WAY TO ORIENT VOLUNTEERS

Volunteers are usually an essential part of the program in a community center, senior citizens' center, or residential facility. You may even be a volunteer yourself. If not, you undoubtedly work with volunteers. If so, it is important to let them know that your center or facility encourages the independence of visually impaired people and takes steps to promote it.

You will want to share with volunteers—and other staff members—the material in earlier chapters of this book. Everyone who works with older people should be familiar with the most common eye conditions; ways in which people adjust to vision loss and in which to be helpful if necessary to visually impaired people; and techniques that can be learned to help people move around, read, write, eat, handle money, and take care of their living quarters and themselves.

Volunteers should also know that negative myths about the helplessness of visually impaired people are just that: myths. You can point out that most people with vision loss can usually function well on their own and have a good deal of remaining vision but that others need some help from people who are concerned about them, such as staff members and volunteers.

To be of assistance, volunteers need to learn some of the things that you have learned. A highly effective way of teaching them is through activities that simulate visual impairment, present problems faced by visually impaired individuals, and demonstrate solutions.

The learning activities that follow are based on the material presented in earlier chapters, so you should review each pertinent chapter with the participants before or while they do an exercise. Bear in mind that these exercises can be used to train staff members, as well as volunteers.

Most of the activities are performed wearing eye masks that simulate visual impairments. The first step in teaching, therefore, is to have the volunteers create simulators for four of the conditions discussed in Chapter 1. They will need to use these simulators for several of the exercises. The patterns to be used appear throughout this chapter, along with a basic blindfold pattern.

Vision Loss Simulators

To make each simulator, first photocopy the pattern. If you have a photocopy machine that will increase the size of copies made, you should check how much larger your simulators might need to be for the people who will be wearing them, and make enlarged copies. If your photocopy machine does not make enlargements, you should check the size you need and make adjustments as you trace and cut your pattern. (Note that the simulators for cataract and diabetic retinopathy are the same pattern; however, different materials are used to simulate the two conditions.)

Then put carbon paper on a piece of poster board, place the photocopy on the carbon paper, and trace the pattern. Cut out the pattern along the solid lines, including the lines for the eye openings. Cut each tab marked down to the dotted line.

Fold down each tab. Overlap the tabs slightly and tape them in place with transparent tape. (Overlapping will hold the simulator off the face a little.) Pierce holes and tie strings to the sides of the simulator.

To complete each simulator, do the following:

- *Age-related maculopathy simulator:* Cut two pieces of clear plastic about an inch larger than the eye opening and glue them to the back. Cut a circle of dark poster board about an inch smaller than the eye opening. Tape the circle to the center of the eye opening so that the person's central vision is blocked off and only a rim of clear plastic remains to see through. When the mask is worn, the peripheral vision caused by age-related maculopathy will be simulated.
- *Cataract simulator:* Crumple and smooth out a small sheet of wax paper. Cut two pieces of wax paper about an inch larger than the eye openings and glue them to the back. When the mask is worn, the general blurring caused by cataracts will be simulated.
- *Diabetic retinopathy simulator*: Cut two pieces of bubble plastic (available in stationery stores) about an inch larger than the eye openings and tape them to the back. Color between the bubbles with black and red indelible markers to give the plastic a spotty appearance.

When the mask is worn, the spotty, blurred vision caused by diabetic retinopathy will be simulated.

- *Glaucoma simulator:* Cut a piece of clear plastic about an inch larger than the small eye opening and glue it to the back. When the mask is worn, the tunnel vision caused by glaucoma will be simulated.

Be sure to have participants mark each mask with the name of the condition it simulates. Now you are ready for the exercises that follow.

Nine Learning Exercises

EXERCISE ONE
DEMONSTRATING WHAT VISUAL IMPAIRMENT FEELS LIKE

Preparation: Set up five tables. On the first table, put a pitcher of water, a glass, and an index card that reads, "Pour water into the glass." On the second table, put a toothbrush, toothpaste, and a card that reads, "Put toothpaste on the toothbrush." On the third table, put some pieces of bread, some butter, knives, and a card that reads, "Butter the bread." On the fourth table, put assorted coins and bills and a card that reads, "Identify the coins and bills." The fifth table should be empty, except for an index card reading, "Take a walk down the hall."

Have the participants, working in pairs, perform the activities requested at each table. While one person wears a simulator, the other monitors his or her progress and safety. Then the participants switch roles. Afterward, they should discuss what it felt like to perform the activities while using the simulators. Solutions to problems caused by lack of vision should be discussed, with an emphasis on how to maintain independence. Then have the participants do the activities again, utilizing the solutions that were presented.

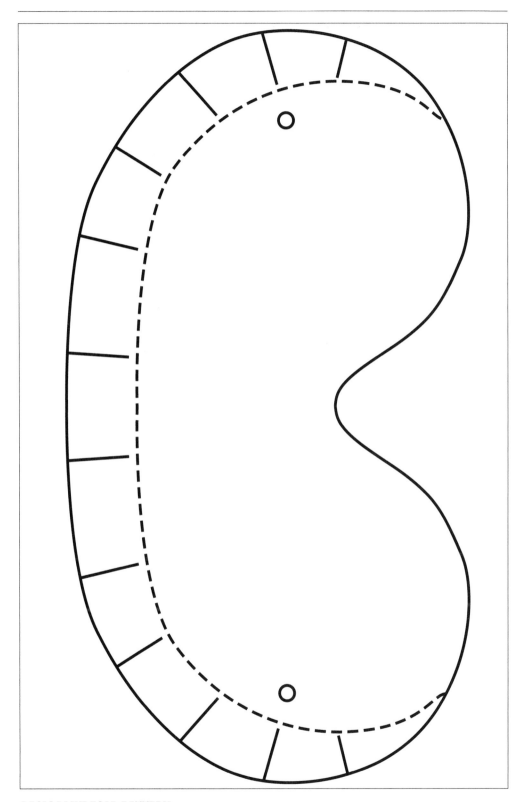

BASIC BLINDFOLD PATTERN.

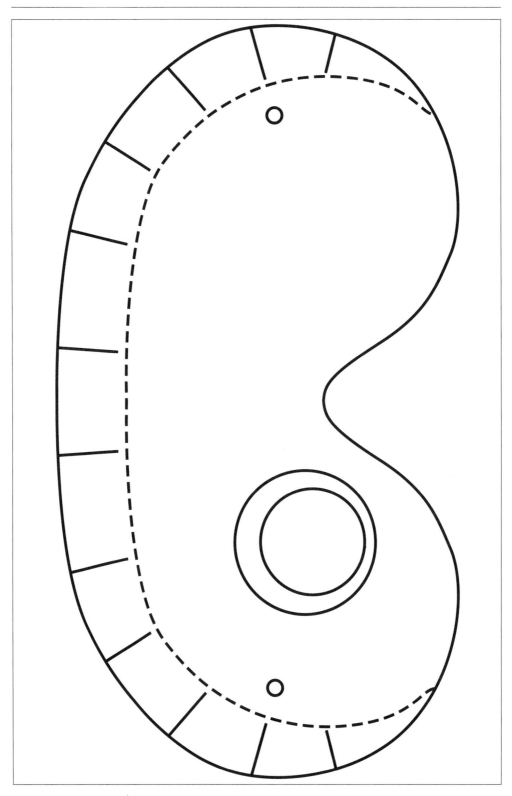

AGE-RELATED MACULOPATHY SIMULATOR.

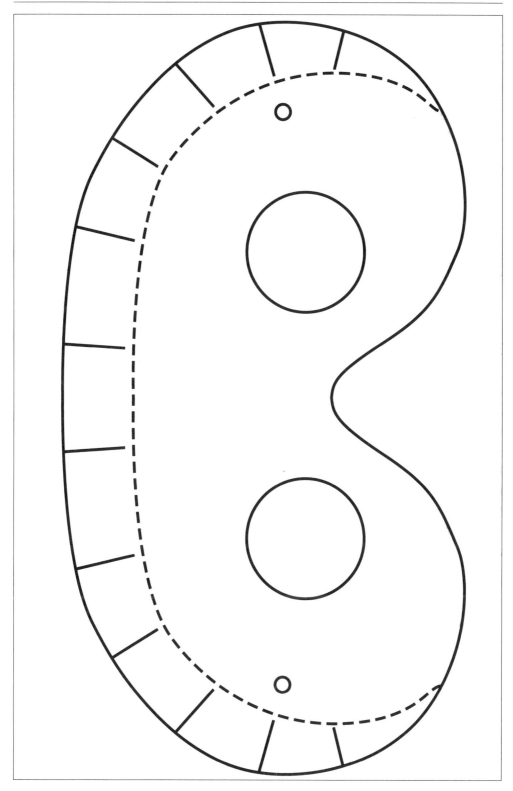

CATARACT SIMULATOR.

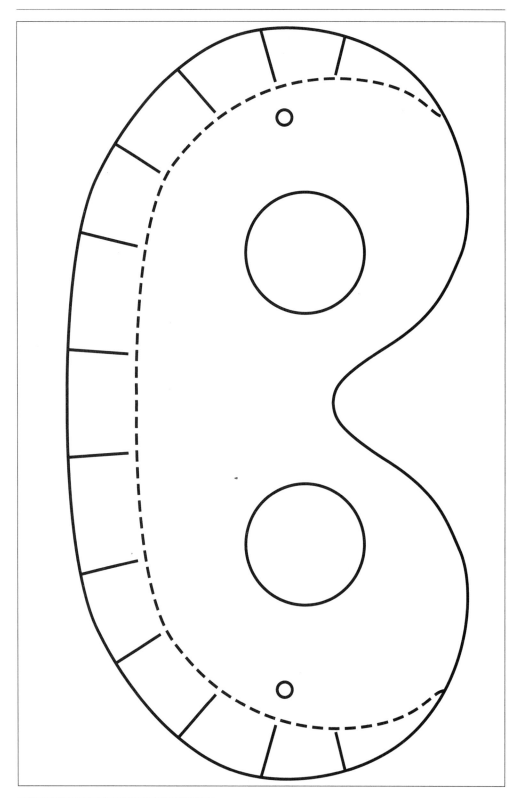

DIABETIC RETINOPATHY SIMULATOR.

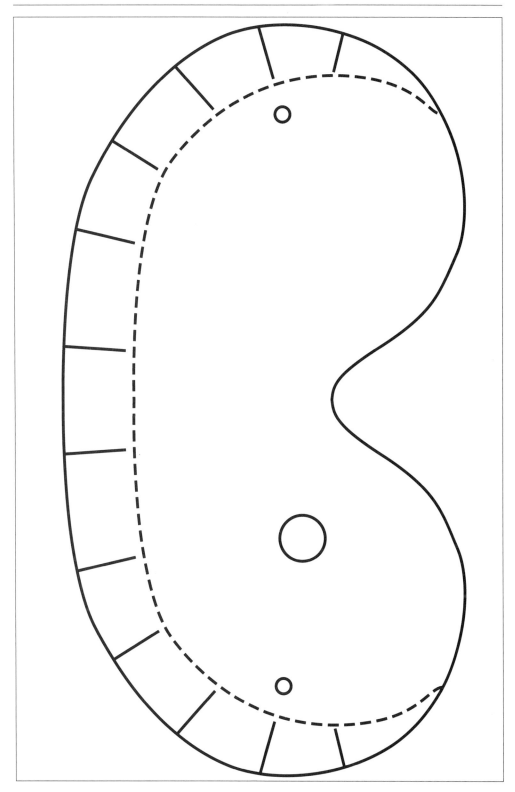

GLAUCOMA SIMULATOR.

EXERCISE TWO
DEMONSTRATING SIGHTED GUIDE TECHNIQUES

Preparation: Set up chairs and tables so there are narrow passageways; chairs at tables; and two rows of chairs simulating seating in an auditorium. If possible, do this exercise where you have access to doorways, a stairway, and a car.

Have the participants, working in pairs, practice the sighted guide techniques described in Chapter 4. Each person should guide and then be guided while wearing a simulator to do the following: navigate a narrow passageway, get seated at a table, get seated in an auditorium, walk down a flight of stairs, and get in and out of a car. Also practice these activities while using support canes; walkers; and, when possible, wheelchairs.

EXERCISE THREE
DEMONSTRATING PROTECTIVE TRAVELING TECHNIQUES

Preparation: Arrange to practice in a common room, a recreation room, or a lounge with a corridor nearby.

As they work in pairs and take turns wearing a simulator, have the participants practice the protective skills presented in Chapter 4—the upper hand and forearm technique, the lower hand and forearm technique, trailing skills, and becoming familiar with a room.

EXERCISE FOUR
DEMONSTRATING READING AIDS

Preparation: On a table, set up a display of the magnifiers and other optical devices described in Chapter 5.

Arrange to have a rehabilitation specialist or some other trained person demonstrate how the devices can be used. Participants should be allowed to handle the devices and look through them.

EXERCISE FIVE
DEMONSTRATING THE USE OF WRITING GUIDES

Preparation: Put a supply of white paper, envelopes, and felt-tip pens on a table. Make enough of the signature guides and envelope guides pictured in Chapter 5 for all the participants. Use card stock or poster board in a dark color, so that the guides contrast with the white paper.

Have each participant clip a signature guide to a piece of paper and an envelope guide to an envelope. Working in pairs, one person should act as a sighted guide, while the other, wearing a simulator, should write a signature and address an envelope. Then the partners should reverse roles.

EXERCISE SIX
DEMONSTRATING EATING TECHNIQUES

Preparation: Put several place settings—a plate, knife, fork, spoon, and water glass—on a table, together with a pitcher of water, a bread basket, a butter dish, and salt and pepper shakers.

Have half the participants wear simulators while the others instruct them in the eating techniques described in Chapter 6. Then have the "students" become the "teachers." During the practice, each person should search to find the drinking glass, learn the clock method for locating food, use a knife to spread butter on the bread, practice pouring water from the pitcher, and add salt and pepper to make-believe "food" on the plate.

EXERCISE SEVEN
DEMONSTRATING HOW TO TELL TIME AND IDENTIFY MONEY

Preparation: Set up two tables. On one, place several envelopes containing assorted bills and coins. On the other table, put a simulated braille clock. If your photocopy machine can make enlargements, you can make the clock by successively enlarging the template shown here until it fits on a piece of poster board 8 1/2 inches by 11 inches. Otherwise, use the template as a model, and draw a circle whose diameter is about 7 1/2 inches, marking off the hours as they are shown on the sample here. Then cut out the clock and glue it to a piece of poster board. Put glue on the dots next to the numbers, and let it dry. Finally, photocopy or draw the hands of the clock and cut them out as well. Attach the hands to the clock with a brass paper fastener.

Have the participants tell time by the braille clock (see Chapter 7). If a braille watch is available, also practice using it.

Then have the participants divide into teams of two and take turns playing the roles of the "sighted" and the "visually impaired" persons. At the money table, one partner folds the bills in the envelopes as described in Chapter 7; then the other partner, wearing a simulator, identifies the bills and the coins. Next, the person wear-

ing the simulator takes bills out of one envelope to make a "purchase," receives change from his or her partner, and folds the bills back into the envelope.

At the time table, the "sighted" person rotates the hands of the clock while the person wearing the simulator tells time by the raised dots.

DEMONSTRATING THE IMPORTANCE OF KEEPING ITEMS ORGANIZED

Preparation: On each of two tables, put small plastic bags and identical collections of personal objects. For example, each collection may have socks; belts; scarves; several pairs of earrings; a toothbrush; toothpaste; and bottles containing hand lotion, shampoo, and liquid soap.

At each table, have a participant wearing a simulator arrange the socks, belts, and scarves according to color; sort the

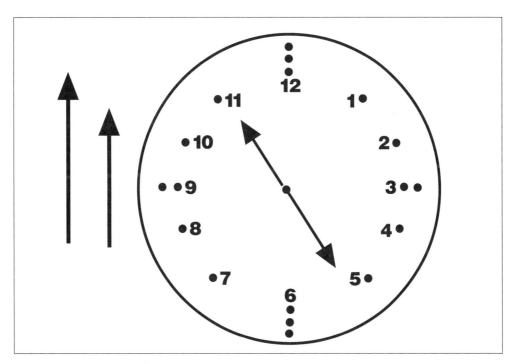

SAMPLE BRAILLE CLOCK.

earrings into plastic bags; and put the bottles near one another—all organizational techniques discussed in Chapter 8. After the organization is completed, ask the two participants to leave the room. While they are gone, rearrange all the items "belonging" to one of them. When the two return, ask them to find the items needed to get ready for a party. Observe that the person whose items were not disturbed has a far easier time.

DEMONSTRATING MENDING AND MEASURING

Preparation: Set up two tables. On one table, place a measuring cup; small bowls; measuring spoons with handles bent to a 90-degree angle; and bottles containing small amounts of water, vinegar, salt, and sugar. On the other table, put needles, a bar of soap to hold the needles, and swatches of light and dark fabric.

Have all participants wear simulators. At the measuring table, have them measure small amounts of liquids and solids into bowls. At the sewing table, have them attempt to thread a needle and sew a few stitches. By doing so, they will be performing two common activities discussed in Chapter 8. In addition, volunteers can also practice sweeping, dusting, and other household tasks, according to the techniques set forth in Chapter 8, while wearing simulators.

Most volunteers find the exercises to be an interesting method of learning about something that is usually new to them. As they put themselves in the place of visually impaired people, they can better relate to the concept of continued independence for every older person. So, by training volunteers, you expand the cadre of people who can offer help in an empathic and effective manner to the visually impaired persons that you know.

CHAPTER 11

DEVELOPING A SUPPORT GROUP

Although most people with visual impairments make their way through life very well, they, like all the rest of us, can sometimes feel alone and worried about the future. They do not realize that others may also have some difficulty doing such things as reading, writing, or managing housework. Although they may confide in you and appreciate your help, they can get a different sort of help from other people who are also visually impaired.

For this reason, it can be valuable to have a support group meet in your senior citizens' center, retirement community, or residential facility. In a well-run group, participants can share common concerns and develop strategies for coping with difficulties. One group member, for example, may know something about vision aids that the others do not know, someone else may have hit upon an easier way of labeling groceries, and so forth. In fact, self-help groups have been found to be a strong and effective way of helping people cope with daily problems.

A group has other purposes, too. It can provide information about the types of resources and services available. It can invite speakers with different areas of expertise. And it can decide to advocate for various legislative measures on behalf of older or visually impaired persons. In short, a support group empowers members by allowing them to make choices about the kind of future they want to have.

Setting a Group Up

With all the knowledge you have gained about helping visually impaired people, you may want to think about starting a self-help group yourself. As with some of the other projects we have discussed in this book, the first step is to discuss the matter with your administrator—unless you are the administrator—and obtain his or her backing.

Once you have done so, you need to find out if there are potential members for the support group. You probably know several visually impaired people to whom you can say something like, "We're thinking of setting up a group where people could meet and talk about living with vision problems. Would you be interested?" You can then describe some of the advantages of such a group.

You can also put a notice on bulletin boards, in the center's or facility's newsletter, in neighboring stores and other buildings, and in the local newspaper. The notice can be as simple as, "Want to join a discussion group for people with vision difficulties?" Put down your name as the contact person and a telephone number or room number at the address where you can be reached.

As people respond, take down their names, addresses, and phone numbers and the times that would be most convenient for them to meet. If possible, choose the time suggested by the majority of respondents. In the case of a senior citizens' center, that may mean a day meeting, since some older people may prefer not to travel extensively at night.

Select the meeting room with care. Look for an accessible place with good lighting, good acoustics, and comfortable seating that will allow the participants to see each other clearly. Some facilities have small lounges that fit this bill. In others, an area in a recreation room or community room may have to be utilized. Make certain that no one else is scheduled to use the room during the time you hold your meeting.

Also exercise care in your choice of a moderator, since this person can be the most important element in a group's success or failure. The moderator should have experience in running support groups and, ideally, a background in counseling, so that he or she can identify people who may need to be referred for individual therapy. If no one in your center or facility has these qualifications, you may be able to find candidates by contacting your state vocational rehabilitation agency or AFB.

Be sure to take plenty of time while interviewing each candidate. Good questions to ask include these: "What do you see as the short-term and long-term goals of a support group?" "How would you involve a group member who hesitates to speak up?" "How would you deal with a person who tends to dominate the group?"

"What types of speakers do you think would be suitable for the group?"

Listen carefully to the responses, and try to imagine the person relating to the visually impaired people you know. You will probably get a sense of who would be "right" for your particular group.

Getting the Group Under Way

Although most decisions will be made by the group, you and the moderator should decide on the time frame. Usually, an hour is ample to allow for the development of issues and a discussion or for a presentation followed by questions.

Before the first meeting, contact everyone who called for information. Ask them to tell friends and neighbors who may also be interested. Do not forget to publicize the meeting on bulletin boards and in newsletters. You may also want to send notices to the nearest low vision centers so they can post them, too.

At the first meeting, you and the moderator should welcome the members and make them feel at home. Discuss the reasons for forming the group.

The first order of business will be for members to decide how often they will meet. They should also formulate ground rules. Here, for example, are some of the rules that groups typically establish:

- Everyone will have the opportunity to talk.
- Members may not walk in and out of the meeting room continually.
- The moderator will telephone members who miss a meeting.

After setting some rules, members will want to talk about topics they may wish to discuss and the formats for presenting them. A mixture of formats is often effective: group discussions, audiovisual presentations, and talks by guest speakers.

Suitable speakers include rehabilitation teachers, O&M specialists, and other experts on living with a visual impairment. You can get referrals for speakers and audiovisual materials from AFB, libraries for visually impaired people, radio reading services, and state and local agencies serving individuals who are visually impaired. Other good sources of materials are distributors of adaptive products (see Resources). Remember, too, that many of the subjects discussed in this book make excellent topics for group meetings.

Making the Group a Success

The success of a support group depends on the enthusiasm of the members, the skills of the moderator, and adherence to time-worn guidelines. Some general principles for making each session go well are found in "Suggestions for Support Group Success."

At the end of meetings, the moderator should make sure to summarize the key points. This is a good way of helping members retain the information. The moderator should also announce the subject of the next meeting and remind everyone to attend. If possible, a notice should be sent out to members before the next meeting.

To stay "healthy" in terms of participation, a group needs to be monitored and worked on. You may want to survey members at regular intervals to find out their reactions. If members are satisfied, ask them to let other visually impaired people know about the group. Post meeting notices on bulletin boards and in appropriate publications. Members who drop out should be contacted by you or the moderator to find out why they no longer attend. Perhaps these people are feeling overlooked, or perhaps the subjects discussed do not interest them. There may be some adjustments you can make to renew their interest.

Finally, remember to give most of the responsibility for the group to the members themselves. The members should

---

SUGGESTIONS FOR SUPPORT GROUP SUCCESS

- Always start and end on time. Put a clock with large numbers at the front of the room.
- Have participants introduce themselves at the beginning of the meeting and say a word or two. This technique serves to draw newcomers into the group.
- Encourage all members to participate in each meeting.
- Allow members to express their feelings in a constructive manner.
- Discourage members from belittling themselves or others. Point out the positives of what they have accomplished.
- Do not allow any one person to monopolize the discussion.
- Discourage conversations between small groups that are not shared with the entire group.
- Be alert for people who may need psychological or medical help.
- Allow plenty of time for questions after a speaker is finished.
- Jot down ideas and questions that emerge from the discussion. If a question cannot be answered, assign someone to explore answers and report on them at the next meeting.
- Keep alert for articles and other publications that should be passed along to the group.

---

be thinking about new subjects, contacting speakers, and opening themselves up to the concerns of others. Ideally, people should grow and acquire confidence from being in the group. When members feel that this is "their place" for sharing problems, developing solutions, and gaining strength, the group becomes a success, and you will know that the effort you put into developing it was worthwhile.

CHAPTER 12

ASSISTANCE FOR FAMILIES

In addition to support groups, families are an important source of support for older people with visual impairments. But in today's world, many families are busy. They may be involved with children and careers and be unaware of a parent's vision problems. Or, they may assume that nothing can be done to make it easier to live with a visual impairment.

As you have learned from reading this book, that is not the case. You know that there are O&M techniques to be used for moving around safely; aids to assist with reading and writing; and adaptive methods for eating, cooking, cleaning, and performing personal grooming tasks. You also know how a visually impaired person's home can be made safer. And you are aware of the services provided by low vision centers, rehabilitation professionals, Talking Book programs, and so forth. You are now in an excellent position to communicate some of what you have learned to families—who need some support themselves if they are to be able to support their visually impaired relatives.

There are several ways to make contact with families. If you have been working closely with a visually impaired individual, ask him or her if you may make an appointment to speak with a family member. The visually impaired person should also attend the meeting, if possible.

At the meeting, try to find out what the family member knows about his or her relative's vision loss. If a vision problem has not yet been diagnosed, but you suspect that one may exist, refer the person and the family member to an ophthalmologist or other eye care specialist or to the nearest low vision center.

If the vision problem is of long standing, determine if the family member understands the ramifications. Does he or she know how vision is affected? What kind of help the relative needs? What types of aids are available? You may want to talk about some of the subjects treated in this book, thereby informing the family member of steps that can be taken to help someone maintain independence. Remember, too, that many of the learning activities outlined in Chapter 10 can be used for teaching families as well as staff and volunteers.

In all your conversations with family members, you should convey a sense of empathy and concern. Just knowing that someone else cares about a parent can make adult children feel less burdened and more receptive to learning what you want to teach about visual impairment.

Keying Families in to Resources

Besides undertaking learning activities and individual conferences, you may want to try these additional ways of reaching out to families:

- Organize meetings with guest speakers who are experts on visual impairment.
- Produce a newsletter on helping visually impaired persons.
- Develop support groups for family members.
- Arrange for demonstrations of products for persons who are visually impaired.

An essential thing you can do is to provide families with a list of local, state, and national agencies serving visually impaired people. For basic information about these agencies and what they do, refer to "Where to Get Help" in Chapter 1 and Resources at the end of this book. If possible, discuss that information with the families you serve.

To create a resource list, use the outline in this chapter. If you wish, make a photocopy of the outline. Then look up the addresses and telephone numbers of local and state agencies and write them in. Finally, make photocopies of the filled-in list and distribute it to the families you work with. It is a good idea, by the way, to keep a copy in your desk, too, and to give copies to other staff members.

The next part of the listing you compile can include a variety of national associations serving visually impaired and older persons, such as the American Council of the Blind (ACB), American Association of Retired Persons (AARP), American Foundation for the Blind (AFB), Blinded Veterans Association (BVA), Library of Congress National Library Service (NLS) for the Blind and Physically Handicapped, National Association of Area Agencies on Aging, National Federation of the Blind (NFB), and National

Society to Prevent Blindness (NSPB). The names, addresses, and telephone numbers of these and other organizations are provided in the Resources section of this book. And the *Directory of Services for Blind and Visually Impaired Persons in the United States and Canada, 24th Edition* (New York: American Foundation for the Blind, 1993) can be consulted for a comprehensive list of such organizations.

Taking an Advocacy Position

Often families and their visually impaired relatives do not know that there are laws protecting people with visual impairments against discrimination. The following is basic information that you can impart about major pieces of legislation.

The Rehabilitation Act of 1973 provides funding to the states for rehabilitation training of visually impaired older adults so that they can remain in their homes. Section 504 of the act mandates that any facility accepting state or federal funds cannot discriminate by not admitting eligible disabled individuals. Under the Omnibus Budget Reconciliation Act of 1987, nursing homes that receive funding from Medicare or Medicaid must maintain residents at optimum levels of independence, functioning, and quality of life. The facility has to show in its records that it is making efforts to achieve these goals.

The Fair Housing Act of 1988 prohibits discrimination in the rental or sale of housing based on disability. The law gives disabled individuals the right to make reasonable modifications in rental apartments at their own expense.

The ADA of 1990, mentioned in Chapter 9, went into effect in January 1992 and has sweeping provisions guaranteeing equal opportunity in employment, public accommodations, transportation, governmental services, long-term care facilities, and retirement centers. It requires that all

RESOURCE LIST FOR FAMILIES

Center or facility name _____

Address _____

Phone No. _____

Contact person _____

There are many agencies available to help you and your visually impaired relative. Here are some names and addresses to keep on hand.

LOCAL AGENCIES

Local agency for visually impaired people

Name _____

Address _____

_____

Phone No. _____

Local agency on aging

Name _____

Address _____

_____

Phone No. _____

Local social services department

Name _____

Address _____

_____

Phone No. _____

Local Social Security Administration office

Name _____

Address _____

_____

Phone No. _____

Local senior citizens' or volunteer center

Name _____

Address _____

_____

Phone No. _____

(continued on next page)

RESOURCE LIST FOR FAMILIES (continued)

Nearest low vision center

Name ______________________________

Address ______________________________

____

Phone No. ______________________________

Nearest library for visually impaired people

Name ______________________________

Address ______________________________

____

Phone No. ______________________________

Radio reading service

Name ______________________________

Address ______________________________

____

Phone No. ______________________________

STATE AGENCIES

State vocational rehabilitation agency

Name ______________________________

Address ______________________________

____

Phone No. ______________________________

State agency for visually impaired people

Name ______________________________

Address ______________________________

____

Phone No. ______________________________

State office on aging

Name ______________________________

Address ______________________________

____

Phone No. ______________________________

places of public accommodation, including residential facilities and social service agencies, such as senior citizens' centers, must remove architectural barriers when removal is readily achievable and, in general, undertake such modifications as are necessary to meet the needs of disabled persons. There are many standards that must be met. Among the regulations that apply to visually impaired people, for example, is one requiring that elevator control buttons be designated both in braille and by raised letters.

Just as important as the many regulations it promulgates is the fact that the act has focused national attention on the rights of disabled people, thus increasing their visibility to the public and their self-esteem. The act gives visually impaired people and their families ammunition with which to fight discrimination. But you can help, too, by taking a strong advocacy position to make sure the law is observed in your center or facility and other environments about which you know. By demonstrating that your center or facility is doing everything it can to support visually impaired people, you can encourage trust by families and also reinforce your own sense of purpose.

CHAPTER 13

THE ISSUE OF RIGHTS

A fitting closing for this book is to talk about how you can further the rights of people who are visually impaired. If you work in a residential setting, you need to be particularly cognizant of this issue, but rights are a valid consideration in other settings as well.

As you know, civil rights legislation—most recently, the ADA—ensures that individuals cannot be discriminated against because they have disabling conditions. Most residential facilities have a bill of rights that informs residents of the right to have privacy, to see their records, to be free of abuse and restraints, to have visitors, to be involved in transfer or discharge planning, to have personal funds safeguarded, and to be protected against discrimination. Many visually impaired people, however, do not understand how these general principles apply to their particular situation. In light of the material discussed in previous chapters, the "bill of rights" included in this chapter considers how the various statements of rights might be interpreted for—and to—visually impaired people, regardless of setting.

In addition to the considerations outlined in this chapter, people should be told that if they think their rights are being violated, they can lodge a complaint with the ombudsperson program, run by the state or local agency for services to aging persons (see "Where to Get Help" in Chapter 1). An ombudsperson is a public official or volunteer who investigates complaints and recommends ways of remedying the situation. The decisions of an ombudsperson are usually binding, and dealing with an ombudsperson is usually easier and more expeditious than filing a complaint of discrimination with a regulatory agency.

It is important to discuss the issue of rights with staff members and volunteers. Rights cannot be safeguarded unless they become part of the consciousness of every person who works with people who are visually impaired. As you can see, they are a natural outgrowth of the subjects we have discussed in this book, a structure that can be used to integrate visually impaired people fully into your program.

A BILL OF RIGHTS FOR PERSONS WITH VISUAL IMPAIRMENTS

1. Upon admission or entrance, people who are visually impaired will be given an orientation tour of the building or facility so they become aware of structural features, landmarks they can use to orient themselves, and potential hazards.

2. People who are visually impaired are entitled to be treated with respect, dignity, and courtesy. They will not be verbally abused or put in restraints or placed on psychoactive drugs in a residential setting because of their visual impairment.

3. Independence, tailored to an individual's level of capability, will be a goal for all persons who are visually impaired. For example, people who can move around the building or facility unaided, take their own medications, and handle their financial and personal affairs will be encouraged to do so. Those who need help in some areas, such as eating, grooming, selecting clothing, or other daily activities, will be offered assistance.

4. People who are visually impaired will be encouraged to participate in a full plan of activities, including outings.

5. People who are visually impaired have the same right to privacy as does anyone else. They will be allowed to arrange their personal possessions, such as toiletries, clothing, and recreational materials, as they see fit, within the bounds of the facility's policy. Housekeeping staff will be told how important it is not to rearrange these items.

6. The environmental needs of people who are visually impaired—such as appropriate lighting and the safe arrangement of furniture—will be taken into consideration. Staff will ask the local agency for visually impaired people for help to correct potential hazards.

7. People who are visually impaired will be alerted to changes in the environment, such as the rearrangement of furniture in common rooms or living quarters, before they take place. Their living quarters will not be rearranged unless it is essential to do so.

8. Written announcements that apply to everyone will be given to persons who are visually impaired in large print or braille or on tape, or they will be read to them by staff members.

9. Staff will inform people who are visually impaired of the specialized services available for them in the community and, if desired, arrange for the use of such services.

GLOSSARY

Acetate sheet. A transparent colored sheet that, when placed over text, reduces glare and makes reading easier for some visually impaired people.

Activities of daily living. Tasks people perform to maintain their health, home, personal appearance, and income. Examples include brushing one's teeth, preparing a meal, mending clothing, and holding down a job.

Adjustment process. The process—consisting of several phases—that a person goes through to cope with the reality of the loss of vision.

Age-related maculopathy. An eye condition that impairs central vision, making it difficult to read, write, or recognize faces. One of the most common eye conditions in older people, it is also called macular degeneration.

Americans with Disabilities Act (ADA). Legislation passed in 1990 that guarantees equal opportunity and access to all disabled citizens, including visually impaired people, in regard to employment, public accommodations, transportation, telecommunications, and governmental services.

Anger and/or withdrawal. A phase in the process of adjustment to visual impairment in which people demonstrate anger, mourn for lost abilities, resent their impairment, and may withdraw from many of their usual activities.

Audiodescription. A taped account describing the visual aspects of and what is happening during a play, television program, or other performance that allows visually impaired persons to follow along.

Cataract. A condition in which the lens of the eye becomes cloudy, thereby blurring the visual field. It can generally be corrected by surgery.

Clock technique. A way of helping visually impaired people to find the food on their plates by referring to the positions of numbers on a clock.

Closed-circuit television (CCTV). A television system that magnifies print so visually impaired people can read more easily.

Color contrast. A way of making objects easier to see by placing light items on or against dark backgrounds, and vice versa.

Coping and mobilization. A phase in the process of adjustment to visual impairment in which the person learns new ways of managing.

Denial. See Shock and denial.

Depression. See Succumbing and depression.

Diabetic retinopathy. An eye condition, affecting people with diabetes, in which damage occurs to the blood vessels behind the eye, resulting in vision loss.

Environmental modifications. Alterations in a home, a facility, or other living quarters that make it easier for visually impaired people to function independently.

Fair Housing Act. Legislation passed in 1988 prohibiting discrimination based on disability in the rental or sale of housing. The law also gives disabled individuals the right to make reasonable modifications in rental apartments at their own expense.

Glaucoma. An eye disease characterized by increased pressure from the buildup of fluid.

Advanced glaucoma can result in tunnel vision or the loss of vision in the peripheral field. If treated early, glaucoma can be controlled by medication.

Hemianopsia. An eye condition, usually caused by a stroke, in which the visual field becomes obstructed.

Labeling. Marking objects with large print, colored markers, or special substances, or in some other way, so they are easily seen by people who are visually impaired.

Legal blindness. The definition of blindness used by the federal government to determine eligibility for certain benefits or services: central visual acuity of 20/200 or less in the better eye with corrective eyeglasses or contact lenses or a visual field of 20 degrees or less.

Library for the visually impaired. A regional library that, under the auspices of the National Library for the Blind and Physically Handicapped, provides taped and other materials to visually impaired people. See also Talking Book Program.

Lighting. The illumination required—in adequate quantities and arrangement—for visually impaired people to read, write, and perform other activities.

Local agency for visually impaired people. An agency that provides a wide range of rehabilitation services and counseling for persons with visual impairments on the local level.

Local agency on aging. An agency that provides services to older adults, such as transportation, telephone contact, home care, escort services, and Meals on Wheels, on the local level.

Local social services department. An agency that provides on the local level general welfare assistance and information on Medicaid, a state-administered medical-assistance program for people whose income and resources fall below a certain level.

Local volunteer center. A local agency that matches volunteers with community projects, including working with or visiting visually impaired people.

Low vision. Vision loss that cannot be corrected to normal by prescribed lenses.

Low vision center. A place where low vision devices are prescribed and specialists provide training in their use, the performance of activities of daily living, and orientation and mobility techniques.

Low vision device. A device such as a magnifier or telescope prescribed by an eye care specialist to enable an individual to make optimum use of remaining vision.

Low vision simulator. A mask that allows the wearer, such as a participant in a training session, to experience the effects of certain eye conditions.

Low vision specialist. A professional, such as an ophthalmologist, optometrist, rehabilitation teacher, or orientation and mobility specialist, who works with visually impaired people in low vision centers.

Lower hand and forearm protective technique. A method used by a visually impaired person to protect the lower body while walking.

Macular degeneration. See Age-related maculopathy.

Milled-edged coin. A coin identifiable by its grooved edges—a dime, a quarter, or a half-dollar.

Mobility. The ability to move from place to place or to move around within an environment.

Mobilization. See Coping and mobilization.

Ombudsperson. A public official or volunteer who, under the auspices of the state agency on aging, investigates grievances from residents against residential facilities, such as nursing homes.

Omnibus Budget Reconciliation Act. Legislation passed in 1987 that establishes standards for the quality of long-term care facilities that receive governmental funding. A facility must maintain residents at optimum levels of independence and functioning.

Ophthalmologist. A physician who specializes in treating people with eye diseases and prescribes eyeglasses, low vision devices, and contact lenses.

Optical aid. A device prescribed by an ophthalmologist or optometrist, such as a magnifier or telescope, that helps visually impaired people to see better.

Optical scanner. A device that reads text aloud in a synthetic voice.

Optician. A technician who fills prescriptions for eyeglasses, contact lenses, and other optical devices and adjusts them as needed.

Optometrist. A professional who specializes in the assessment and treatment of visual problems and prescribes eyeglasses, low vision optical devices, and contact lenses.

Orientation. Use of the senses to determine where one is and the direction in which one is traveling.

Orientation and mobility specialist. A professional who teaches visually impaired people how to move around safely with the use of special techniques.

Personal care techniques. Methods used by visually impaired people to perform such activities as bathing, dressing, or brushing teeth.

Radio reading service. A radio station specializing in the broadcast of books, magazines, and other reading materials to visually impaired subscribers. Most states have at least one such station.

Reassessment and reaffirmation. A phase of the adjustment process to visual impairment in which people identify their strengths and start to plan for the future.

Rehabilitation Act of 1973. Federal legislation that provides for rehabilitation training, including the training of visually impaired people.

Rehabilitation teacher. A professional who teaches visually impaired people how to perform activities of daily living safely and efficiently.

Rheostat. An electrical device for regulating the degree of lighting in a room.

Room-familiarization technique. A method that visually impaired people can learn to explore a room that is new to them.

Shock and denial. A phase in the process of adjustment to visual impairment in which people deny that they are losing their vision.

Sighted guide technique. A technique that a person who is not visually impaired can use to help a person with vision loss move safely from place to place.

Smooth-edged coin. A coin identifiable by its smooth edges—a penny or nickel.

State office on aging. An agency that funds programs, carried out by local offices on aging, to serve older adults in a state. It also provides for a long-term-care ombudsperson program. See also Ombudsperson.

State vocational rehabilitation agency. An agency that provides counseling, low vision services, rehabilitation services, and vocational services in a state, often through local agencies for visually impaired people.

Succumbing and depression. A phase of the adjustment process to visual impairment in which the person exhibits strong grief reactions.

Talking Book Program. A service, available through the National Library for the Blind and Physically Handicapped, that provides taped materials to people who are visually impaired and physically handicapped. See also Library for the visually impaired.

Trailing. A technique used by visually impaired people for getting around safely. It involves moving the fingertips along a wall or some other surface to keep a straight line, to find an object, or to orient oneself to an area.

Trauma. A phase in the adjustment process to visual impairment in which a person experiences extreme stress or dismay as a result of the diagnosis.

Upper hand and forearm protective technique. A method used by a visually impaired person to protect the upper part of the body while walking.

Visual impairment. Vision loss that interferes with the performance of certain activities of daily living.

Withdrawal. See Anger and/or withdrawal.

Writing guide. A template—cutout pattern—used to assist visually impaired people in signing their names or addressing envelopes.

RESOURCES

RESOURCES

A wide variety of organizations and companies disseminate information, distribute adaptive equipment, and provide various forms of assistance to people who are blind or visually impaired, their families, and the professionals who work with them. This section contains a sample listing of these organizations and companies. Additional information can be found in the *Directory of Services for Blind and Visually Impaired Persons in the United States and Canada, 24th Edition*, published by the American Foundation for the Blind.

NATIONAL ORGANIZATIONS

American Association of Retired Persons
601 E Street, N.W.
Washington, DC 20049
(202) 434-2277

The American Association of Retired Persons (AARP) is a consumer organization that serves its membership of older Americans by offering a range of community services and educational programs, including technical assistance on legal issues, insurance, and a wide variety of consumer products and other benefits. AARP also disseminates information on consumer affairs; health, financial, and disability issues; and advocacy and publishes *Modern Maturity*.

American Council of the Blind
1155 15th Street, N.W., Suite 720
Washington, DC 20005
(202) 467-5081 or (800) 424-8666

The American Council of the Blind (ACB) is a consumer organization that promotes effective participation of blind and visually impaired people in all aspects of society. It provides information and referral, legal assistance, scholarships, advocacy, consultation services, and program development assistance, and publishes *The Braille Forum*.

American Foundation for the Blind
15 West 16th Street
New York, NY 10011
(212) 620-2000 or (800) 232-5463

The American Foundation for the Blind (AFB) provides a wide variety of services to and acts as an information clearinghouse for people who are blind or visually impaired and their families, professionals, organizations, schools, and corporations. It conducts information and educational programs; provides consultative services; stimulates research to improve services to visually impaired persons; sells adaptive products; advocates for services and legislation; produces videos; and publishes books, pamphlets, the *Directory of Services for Blind and Visually Impaired Persons in the United States and Canada,* and the *Journal of Visual Impairment & Blindness.* AFB maintains the following regional centers across the country, as well as a governmental relations department in Washington, DC:

AFB Resource Center
100 Peachtree Street, Suite 620
Atlanta, GA 30303
(404) 525-2303

Serves Georgia, Puerto Rico, and the Virgin Islands.

Eastern Regional Center
1615 M Street, N.W., Suite 250
Washington, DC 20036
(202) 457-1487

Serves Connecticut, Delaware, District of Columbia, Maine, Maryland, Massachusetts, New Hampshire, New Jersey, New York, North Carolina, Pennsylvania, Rhode Island, South Carolina, Vermont, and Virginia.

Midwest Regional Center
401 North Michigan Avenue, Suite 308
Chicago, IL 60611
(312) 245-9961
Serves Illinois, Indiana, Iowa, Kentucky, Michigan, Minnesota, Missouri, North Dakota, Ohio, South Dakota, Tennessee, West Virginia, and Wisconsin.

Southwest Regional Center
260 Treadway Plaza
Exchange Park
Dallas, TX 75235
(214) 352-7222
Serves Alabama, Arkansas, Colorado, Florida, Kansas, Louisiana, Mississippi, Montana, Nebraska, New Mexico, Oklahoma, Texas, and Wyoming.

Western Regional Center
111 Pine Street, Suite 725
San Francisco, CA 94111
(415) 392-4845
Serves Alaska, Arizona, California, Guam, Hawaii, Idaho, Nevada, Oregon, Utah, and Washington.

American National Standards Institute
655 15th Street, N.W., Suite 300
Washington, DC 20005
(202) 639-4090
The American National Standards Institute (ANSI) provides information about the standards for creating accessible environments for people with disabilities.

Association for Macular Diseases
210 East 64th Street
New York, NY 10021
(212) 605-3719
The Association for Macular Diseases is a consumer organization that provides information and educational services, sponsors support groups for persons with macular degeneration, funds an eye bank devoted to research on macular degeneration, offers individual and group counseling, and publishes a newsletter.

Association of Radio Reading Services
c/o Radio Information Service
2100 Wharton Street, Suite 140
Pittsburgh, PA 15230
(412) 388-3944
The Association of Radio Reading Services promotes radio reading services throughout the United States. It provides closed-circuit radio broadcasts of daily newspapers and other materials, maintains a circulating library of books and programs on tape, and publishes *Hearsay Newsletter* and the *Directory of Radio Reading Services.*

Blinded Veterans Association
477 H Street, N.W.
Washington, DC 20001-2694
(202) 371-8880 or (800) 669-7079
The Blinded Veterans Association (BVA) encourages and assists blind and visually impaired veterans to take advantage of rehabilitation and vocational training benefits, job placement services, and other aid from federal, state, and local resources. Through its regional groups and field service offices, BVA also operates a volunteer service program for blind veterans in their communities, provides information and referral services, and promotes legislation that benefits blind veterans.

Council of Citizens with Low Vision International
5707 Brockton Drive, Suite 302
Indianapolis, IN 46220-5481
(317) 638-6555 or (800) 773-2258
The Council of Citizens with Low Vision International (CCLV) is a consumer organization that promotes the rights of visually impaired persons to maximize the use of their remaining vision. CCLV educates the public about the needs of visually impaired

persons, informs persons of available services, operates support groups and chapters through the United States, and publishes *CCLV News.*

Delta Gamma Foundation
3250 Riverside Drive
P.O. Box 21397
Columbus, OH 43221-0397
(614) 481-8169

The Delta Gamma Foundation provides services to blind and visually impaired persons through cooperation with local agencies; conducts the Delta Gamma Project on Sight Conservation and Aid to the Blind; provides a means for its members to further charitable, scientific, and educational objectives; and publishes *Anchora of Delta Gamma* and *Shield.*

Library of Congress
National Library Service for the Blind and Physically Handicapped
1291 Taylor Street, N.W.
Washington, DC 20542
(202) 707-5100 or (800) 424-8567

The Library of Congress National Library Service(NLS) for the Blind and Physically Handicapped conducts a national program that distributes free reading materials to individuals who cannot use ordinary printed materials because of a visual or physical impairment. It also provides a reference information service on all aspects of blindness and other disabilities that affect reading, conducts national correspondence courses to train sighted persons as braille transcribers and blind persons as braille proofreaders, transcribes books into braille, records books on tape, and repairs special playback equipment for its tapes.

National Association of Area Agencies on Aging
1112 16th Street, N.W., Suite 100
Washington, DC 20036
(202) 296-8130

The National Association of Area Agencies on Aging acts as a national advocate to effect changes that will benefit older persons. It also disseminates information to the federal government, other national organizations, and the public and publishes the *Directory of State and Area Agencies on Aging.*

National Federation of the Blind
1800 Johnson Street
Baltimore, MD 21230
(410) 659-9314

The National Federation of the Blind (NFB) is a consumer organization that strives to improve the social and economic conditions of blind persons, evaluates and assists in establishing programs, and provides public education and scholarships. It also publishes *The Braille Monitor* and *Future Reflections.*

National Society to Prevent Blindness
500 East Remington Road
Schaumburg, IL 60173
(708) 843-2020 or (800) 221-3004

The National Society to Prevent Blindness (NSPB) conducts a program of public and professional education, research, and industrial and community services to prevent blindness. Its services include the promotion and support of local glaucoma and preschool vision screening programs and of industrial eye safety programs, the collection of data on the nature and extent of causes of blindness and visual impairment, and the promotion of improved environmental conditions affecting eye health in schools and colleges. It also publishes *Prevent Blindness News* and *Sightsaving.*

SOURCES OF PRODUCTS AND ADAPTIVE EQUIPMENT
The organizations and companies listed here carry a wide variety of products, including independent living, health care, and recreation products; low vision devices; and communication aids. Products can sometimes be ordered by catalog, which can be obtained from the individual organizations listed.

Aids Unlimited
1101 North Calvert Street
Baltimore, MD 21202
(301) 659-0232

American Foundation for the Blind
Product Center
3342 Melrose Avenue
Roanoke, VA 24107
(800) 829-0500

Ann Morris Enterprises
890 Fams Court
East Meadow, NY 11554
(516) 292-9232

Carolyn's Catalog
17355 Mierow Lane
Brookfield, WI 53045
(800) 648-2266

HumanWare
6245 King Road
Loomis, CA 95650
(916) 652-7253 or (800) 722-3393

Independent Living Aids
27 East Mall
Plainview, NY 11803
(516) 752-8080 or (800) 537-2118

The Lighthouse
36-02 Northern Boulevard
Long Island City, NY 11101
(718) 937-9338 or (800) 453-4923

LS&S Group
P.O. Box 673
Northbrook, IL 60065
(708) 498-9777 or (800) 468-4789

Maxi-Aids
42 Executive Boulevard
P.O. Box 3209
Farmingdale, NY 11735
(516) 752-0521 or (800) 522-6294

National Federation of the Blind
1800 Johnson Street
Baltimore, MD 21230
(301) 659-9314

Seeing Technologies
7074 Brooklyn Boulevard
Minneapolis, MN 55429
(612) 560-8080

TeleSensory Corporation
455 North Bernardo Avenue
P.O. Box 7455
Mountain View, CA 94039-7455
(415) 960-0920 (voice/TDD) or
(800) 227-8418 (voice/TDD)

PRINT AND TAPED MATERIALS AND FILMS

Although the materials listed here are grouped according to chapter as chapter references and for the reader's convenience, they may be generally helpful and relate to the subjects of more than one chapter and to the overall issue of living with vision loss in later life. Their availability at the time of writing is also indicated; local public libraries may, in addition, be sources of some of these materials.

CHAPTER 1

AFB directory of services for blind and visually impaired persons in the United States and Canada, 24th edition (book). (1993). State-by-state listings of agencies and other resources available for visually impaired people. Available from American Foundation for the Blind, c/o American Book Center, Brooklyn Navy Yard, Building No. 3, Brooklyn, NY 11205; (718) 852-9873.

Age-related sensory changes: An empathetic approach (film). Shows how visual conditions affect elderly persons and what can be done to assist in adjustment. Available from University of Michigan Media Resource Center, 416 Fourth Street, Ann Arbor, MI 48109; (313) 764-5360. Rental or purchase.

Aging and vision: Making the most of impaired vision (brochure). (1987). Reviews the major causes of visual impairment in older adults and provides tips on ways to make homes safer. Available from

American Foundation for the Blind, c/o American Book Center, Brooklyn Navy Yard, Building No. 3, Brooklyn, NY 11205; (718) 852-9873.

Aston, S., DeSylvia, D., & Mancil, G. **Optometric gerontology** (book). (1989). A training curriculum on aging and vision. Available from Association of Schools and Colleges of Optometry, 6110 Executive Boulevard, Suite 514, Rockville, MD 20852; (301) 231-5944.

Aston, S., Lepri, B., & Smith, A. **Vision of older persons workshop** (book). (1987). A workshop on vision loss for those who work with older people. Available from Pennsylvania College of Optometry, 1200 West Godfrey Avenue, Philadelphia, PA 19141; (215) 276-6291.

Beliveau, T., & Duffy, M. **New independence: Caring for older visually impaired residents in a nursing home** (book). (1991). A curriculum for nursing home staff that explains eye diseases and presents tips on caring for visually impaired elderly people. Available from AWARE, P.O. Box 96, Mohegan Lake, NY 10547; (914) 528-0567.

A better view of you (slide program-cassettes). Illustrates the functional implications of eye diseases. Available from the Lighthouse, National Center for Vision and Aging, 800 Second Avenue, New York, NY 10017; (212) 808-0077. Purchase or rental.

Caring for nursing home residents with impaired vision (videotape). Explains eye diseases, their functional implications, and adaptive techniques. Available from Rehabilitation Research and Development Center, VAMC, MS-153, 1670 Clairmont Road, Decatur, GA 30033; (404) 321-5828.

Jose, R. (Ed.) **Understanding low vision** (book). (1983). Discusses optics, eye diseases, assessment procedures, services, training, and aids. Available from American Foundation for the Blind, c/o American Book Center, Brooklyn Navy Yard, Building No. 3, Brooklyn, NY 11205; (718) 852-9873

Low vision questions and answers: Definitions, devices, services (brochure). (1987). Defines the term *low vision* and tells where to get services and aids. Available from American Foundation for the Blind, c/o American Book Center, Brooklyn Navy Yard, Building No. 3, Brooklyn, NY 11205; (718) 852-9873.

Not without sight (videotape). Depicts the major types of visual impairment and demonstrates how remaining vision can be utilized. Available from American Foundation for the Blind, c/o American Book Center, Brooklyn Navy Yard, Building No. 3, Brooklyn, NY 11205; (718) 852-9873.

A photographic essay on partial sight (poster). Shows scenes of the way a person with visual impairment would see them and describes treatment options. Available from Lighthouse Low Vision Products, 36-02 Northern Boulevard, Long Island City, NY 11101; (800) 453-4923.

Referring blind and low vision patients for rehabilitation services: A guide for ophthalmologists (brochure). (1986). A review of available services. Available from American Foundation for the Blind, c/o American Book Center, Brooklyn Navy Yard, Building No. 3, Brooklyn, NY 11205; (718) 852-9873.

Van Son, A. **Diabetes, vision impairment, and blindness** (brochure). (1985). Explains how diabetes can affect vision and provides techniques for maintaining independence. Available from American Foundation for the Blind, c/o American Book Center, Brooklyn Navy Yard, Building No. 3, Brooklyn, NY 11205; (718) 852-9873.

CHAPTER 2

Look out for Annie (videotape). Depicts an older woman's loss of vision, her psychological reactions, and the rehabilitative services she received. Available from the Lighthouse, 800 Second Avenue, New York, NY 10017; (212) 808-0077.

Ludwig, I., Luxton, L., & Attmore, M. *Creative recreation for blind and visually impaired adults* (book). (1988). Shows how hobbies, sports, and other leisure-time pursuits can be adapted to the needs and abilities of visually impaired persons. Available from American Foundation for the Blind, c/o American Book Center, Brooklyn Navy Yard, Building No. 3, Brooklyn, NY 11205; (718) 852-9873.

Orr, A. *Vision and aging: Crossroads for service delivery* (book). (1992). A comprehensive discussion of the physiological and psychological effects of aging and vision loss. Also includes an overview of current social services. Available from American Foundation for the Blind, c/o American Book Center, Brooklyn Navy Yard, Building No. 3, Brooklyn, NY 11205; (718) 852-9873.

Ringgold, N. *Out of the corner of my eye* (book). (1991). An 87-year-old woman, a former college professor, tells the moving story of her adjustment to vision loss and provides practical advice and cheerful encouragement. Available from American Foundation for the Blind, c/o American Book Center, Brooklyn Navy Yard, Building No. 3, Brooklyn, NY 11205; (718) 852-9873.

Tuttle, D. *Self-esteem and adjusting with blindness* (book). (1984). Describes the phases of adjustment to vision loss and provides coping strategies for each one. Available from Charles C Thomas, 2600 South First Street, Springfield, IL 62717.

CHAPTER 3

A picture is worth a thousand words for blind and visually impaired persons too! An introduction to audiodescription (brochure). (1991). Presents the basic aspects of audiodescription—

the art of verbally describing the visual aspects of a performance. Includes an extensive resource section. Available from American Foundation for the Blind, c/o American Book Center, Brooklyn Navy Yard, Building No. 3, Brooklyn, NY 11205; (718) 852-9873.

What do you do when you see a blind person? (And what you don't do) (brochure). Suggests appropriate ways to communicate with people who are visually impaired. Presented in a cartoon format. Available from American Foundation for the Blind, c/o American Book Center, Brooklyn Navy Yard, Building No. 3, Brooklyn, NY 11205; (718) 852-9873.

CHAPTER 4

The seven-minute lesson (16mm film and videotape). A brief introduction to sighted-guide technique. Available from American Foundation for the Blind, c/o American Book Center, Brooklyn Navy Yard, Building No. 3, Brooklyn, NY 11205; (718) 852-9873.

Welsh, R. L., & Blasch, B. B. *Foundations of orientation and mobility* (book). (1980). The history, theory, and practice of orientation and mobility. Available from American Foundation for the Blind, c/o American Book Center, Brooklyn Navy Yard, Building No. 3, Brooklyn, NY 11205; (718) 852-9873.

CHAPTER 5

Bailey, I. L., & Hall, A. *Visual impairment: An overview* (book). (1990). Presents an overview of eye disease and discusses technology for reading. Available from American Foundation for the Blind, c/o American Book Center, Brooklyn, NY 11205; (718) 852-9873.

Dickman, I. R. (1983). *Making life more livable* (book). (1983). Describes and pictures adaptations for living with visual impairment, including techniques for writing more efficiently. Available from American Foundation for the Blind, c/o American Book Center, Brooklyn Navy Yard, Building No. 3, Brooklyn, NY 11205; (718) 852-9873.

Greenblatt, S. *Providing services for people with vision loss* (book). (1989). An overview of services, including information on communication aids for reading and writing. Available from Resources for Rehabilitation, 33 Bedford Street, Suite 19A, Lexington, MA 02173; (617) 862-6455.

CHAPTER 6

Dickman, I. R. *Making life more livable* (see listings for Chapter 5).

Yeadon, A. *Toward independence: The use of instructional objectives in teaching daily living skills to the blind* (book). (1974). A task-oriented approach to teaching activities of daily living. Available from American Foundation for the Blind, c/o American Book Center, Brooklyn Navy Yard, Building No. 3, Brooklyn, NY 11205; (718) 852-9873.

CHAPTER 7

Caring for the visually impaired older person (book). (1970). Describes techniques for telling time and identifying coins and bills. Available from the Minneapolis Society for the Blind, 1936 Lyndale Avenue South, Minneapolis, MN 55403; (612) 871-2222.

Dickman, I. R. *Making life more livable* (see listings for Chapter 5).

Ringgold, N. *Out of the corner of my eye* (see listings for Chapter 2).

CHAPTER 8

Aging and vision: Making the most of impaired vision (brochure) (see listings for Chapter 1).

Dickman, I. R. *Making life more livable* (see listings for Chapter 5).

A step-by-step guide to personal management for blind persons (book, 2nd ed). (1974). A task-analysis approach to activities of daily living. Available from American Foundation for the Blind, c/o American Book Center, Brooklyn Navy Yard, Building No. 3, Brooklyn, NY 11205; (718) 852-9873.

A vision of independence (videotape). Tells family members how to use lighting, color contrast, and appropriate modifications to make the homes of visually impaired relatives safer. Available from Rehabilitation Research and Development Center, VAMC, MS-153, 1670 Clairmont Road, Decatur, GA 30033; (404) 321-5828. Purchase.

CHAPTER 9

Crews, J. "Strategic planning and independent living for elders who are blind" (article). (1991, May). *Journal of Visual Impairment & Blindness, 85*, 52-58. Presents statistics and makes recommendations for planning services. Available from *Journal of Visual Impairment & Blindness*, c/o Boyd Printing, 49 Sheridan Avenue, Albany, NY 12210; (800) 877-2693.

Kirchner, C. (1988). *Data on blindness and visual impairment in the U.S.* (book). (1988). Data that can be used for long-range planning, preparation of grant proposals, and supporting advocacy positions. Available from American Foundation for the Blind, c/o American Book Center, Brooklyn Navy Yard, Building No. 3, Brooklyn, NY 11205; (718) 852-9873.

Orr, A. *Vision and aging: Crossroads for service delivery* (see listings for Chapter 2).

The unexpected fall (videotape). Safety techniques, designed for use with people who have Alzheimer's disease, that can also be used to protect visually impaired older people. Available from the Alzheimer's Association, 3120 Raymond Drive, Atlanta, GA 30340; (404) 451-1300. Rental.

CHAPTER 10

Franks, J. (1986, March). "A program for sighted, blind, low vision, and disabled volunteers" (article). *Journal of Visual Impairment & Blindness, 80*, 631-32. Reviews the structure of a volunteer program serving blind and visually impaired people. Available from *Journal of Visual Impairment & Blindness*, c/o Boyd Printing, 49 Sheridan Avenue, Albany, NY 12210; (800) 877-2693.

Low vision simulators (kit). Simulators of various types of vision loss and visual acuity ranges. Available from Dr. George Zimmerman, 1932 Woodside Road, Glenshaw, PA 15116-2113; (412) 487-2818.

Wilson, M. *The effective management of volunteer programs* (book). (1976). Describes how to organize and maintain a volunteer program in a facility. Stresses effective communication skills. Available from Volunteer Management Associates, 1113 Spruce Street, Suite 406, Boulder, CO 80302; (303) 447-0558.

Wilson, M. *Survival skills for managers* (book). (1982). Gives managers of volunteer programs information on fostering creativity, problem solving, conflict resolution, stress reduction, time management, and other skills. Available from Volunteer Management Associates, 1113 Spruce Street, Suite 406, Boulder, CO 80302; (303) 447-0558.

CHAPTER 11

Aging and vision: Declarations of independence (videotape). A look at five senior citizens who have overcome their recent vision loss to lead active lives. Available from American Foundation for the Blind, c/o American Book Center, Brooklyn Navy Yard, Building No. 3, Brooklyn, NY 11205; (718) 852-9873.

Poison ivy (videotape). A 66-year-old woman enjoys life despite her visual impairment. Available from Phoenix Films, 468 Park Avenue South, New York, NY 10016; (212) 684-5910. Purchase.

To share a vision (videotape). The main character discovers his visual impairment and comes to accept it. Available from Phoenix Films, 468 Park Avenue South, New York, NY 10016; (212) 684-5910. Purchase.

CHAPTER 12

AFB directory of services for blind and visually impaired persons in the United States and Canada, 24th edition (see listings for Chapter 1).

Awareness is the first step towards change: The Americans with Disabilities Act (brochure). An overview of the act. Available at no charge from the National Easter Seals Society, 70 East Lake Street, Chicago, IL 60601; (312) 726-6200.

Information on the Americans with Disabilities Act (brochure). Describes the provisions of the act. Available at no charge from the Americans with Disabilities Act Enforcement Section, Civil Rights Division, U.S. Department of Justice, P.O. Box 66118, Washington, DC 20035-6118.

Low vision questions and answers: Definitions, devices, services (see listings for Chapter 1).

Tuttle, D. *Self-esteem and adjusting with blindness* (see listings for Chapter 2).

Watson, G., Ernst, S., & Blair, J. *Family training program in low vision curriculum* (book). (1990). A resource list of aids, devices, films, and videotapes in the area of visual impairment. Available from the Rehabilitation Research and Development Center, VAMC, MS-153, 1670 Clairmont Road, Decatur, GA 30033; (404) 321-5828.

ABOUT THE AUTHORS

Nora Griffin-Shirley, Ph.D., is assistant professor and coordinator, orientation and mobility program, Texas Tech University, Lubbock, Texas, and was previously regional consultant in aging, American Foundation for the Blind Southeast Regional Center, Atlanta, Georgia. As an orientation and mobility specialist for visually impaired persons, she has worked extensively with older adults with visual impairments and contributed to the development of a curriculum on aging and vision loss for university gerontology programs, *Aging and Vision Loss: Guidelines for an Innovative Personnel Preparation Curriculum in Gerontology.* Named the Outstanding Graduate Student of the Year at Georgia State University's Gerontology Program in 1990 and the recipient of the Retirement Research Foundation National Media Award for the training videotape *Caring for Nursing Home Residents with Impaired Vision,* she has made numerous presentations on aging and blindness both nationally and internationally.

Gerda Groff, M.Ed., is an educator teaching in Atlanta, Georgia, and was previously regional director, American Foundation for the Blind Southeast Regional Center in Atlanta. The author of *What Museum Guides Need to Know: Access for Blind and Visually Impaired Visitors,* she has provided public education services, consultation, and training to schools, museums, agencies, and community organizations on a wide variety of topics related to vision loss.

THE MISSION of the American Foundation for the Blind (AFB) is to enable persons who are blind or visually impaired to achieve equality of access and opportunity that will ensure freedom of choice in their lives.

∞

It is the policy of the American Foundation for the Blind to use in the first printing of its books acid-free paper that meets the ANSI Z39.48 Standard. The infinity symbol that appears above indicates that the paper in this printing meets that standard.